First Steps in
Veterinary Science

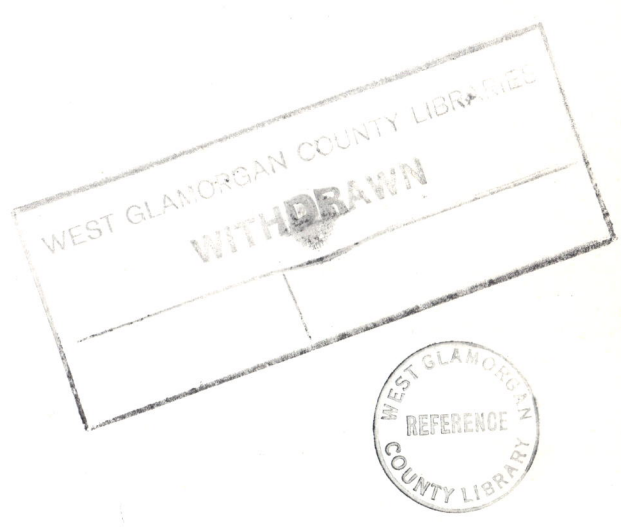

First Steps in Veterinary Science

K. W. ASPINALL MRCVS

*Research Officer (Veterinary Sciences), Central
Veterinary Laboratory, Weybridge, England
Formerly Director of Veterinary Services and
Animals Industry, Malawi*

kenneth

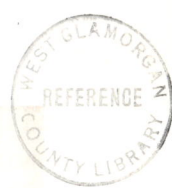

BAILLIÈRE TINDALL   LONDON

A BAILLIÈRE TINDALL book published by
Cassell & Collier Macmillan Publishers Ltd
35 Red Lion Square, London WC1R 4SG
and at Sydney, Auckland, Toronto, Johannesburg
an affiliate of
Macmillan Publishing Co. Inc.
New York

© 1976 Baillière Tindall
a division of Cassell & Collier Macmillan Publishers Ltd

First published 1976

ISBN 0 7020 0635 1

Printed in Great Britain at The Spottiswoode Ballantyne Press,
by William Clowes & Sons Limited,
London, Colchester and Beccles

Contents

Preface

Veterinary work is universal in its application. Causes of disease may differ in accordance with the climate, the environment and the geographical location of the animals, but biological factors which determine an animal's response to hazards remain the same.

The intention of this book is to provide a background of information on which the reader may build. The lay-out of the chapters arose from experience of working with technical assistants over many years in practical conditions of disease control, animal management, animal treatment and animal production. It owes a great deal to contact and discussion with other working veterinarians in tropical and temperate parts of the world. It is hoped that it will enable the technical assistant in training to grasp the essentials of the craft he is acquiring, while relying upon his teacher to expand upon matters discussed. The book should be of value to the agricultural student seeking to grasp the basis of animal husbandry and will also give some indication of just what is meant by veterinary work to those considering a career among animals. Some of the illustrations will be strange to European readers, but Zebu cattle are probably more widely distributed and more numerous throughout the world than temperate breeds.

The book was based upon one designed overseas at a difficult time, and for which there were a number of contributors. It is not possible to acknowledge all who have helped and encouraged its further development, except to thank those who have worked with the author in many capacities during his diverse career. The practical help of the Commonwealth Veterinary Association is also remembered with gratitude, as are those veterinarians in the United Kingdom who have read the script and made their comments.

August 1976 K. W. Aspinall

Introduction

MAN AND ANIMALS—THEIR INTER-RELATIONSHIP

Man has been called the only carnivorous primate, but it is quite clear that he is not an exclusive eater of animal protein. Indeed it seems very probable that he evolved from creatures which ate any food material that they could find. Scavenging for vegetable and insect food is a very time-consuming occupation; and it is reasonable to suppose that early man-like creatures first ate the leavings of specialized carnivores like the big cats, and then learnt to kill for themselves. In order to kill ever more efficiently and to reach animals which would otherwise have eluded him, man gradually evolved the use of weapons; in all probability the club and the spear came first. Once he had food in plenty, he experimented with skins for clothing and bones for weapons and tools.

The domestication of animals is a very much more recent phenomenon. One must conclude that as man learnt to kill animals with greater efficiency his food source became more assured, and he was able not only to extend his hunting range but to expand in numbers. Starvation still imposes the greatest control on animal as well as human populations. There must have come a time when hunting was difficult and some local innovator decided to herd animals against the seasons when meat was hardest to come by. It would seem that the bovine was his first choice and sheep and goats came rather later. Horses were only domesticated in numbers when cereals had been planted and their use in war by armed nomads seeking grains stored in villages had been demonstrated. Pigs were probably domesticated in the vicinity of the great forests.

The inter-relationships between man and animals are still expanding. More and more meat is eaten by a rapidly increasing human population, not only because it is highly nutritious but because people like it. Despite the prevalence of man-made fibres there is still a great demand for animal skins, hair and wool. The most astonishing expansion of the relationship has, however, been in connection with the companion animal. Dogs and cats have always been kept by prosperous human communities for the social comfort they can provide, and horses have become the leisure animal *par excellence*. There is also increasing interest in game animals.

Oxen, horses, camels, and donkeys have long been of importance as transport and traction animals. They are still eminently suited for this purpose in many parts of the world, and it is probable that they have never been so numerous.

It is obvious that man's basic relationship with animals is a utilitarian one. They are needed for food, clothing, traction or transport; in the case of dogs for protection, and in the case of cats for rodent control. As human populations increase and become more densely packed into towns, so does the processing of animals become more organized or industrialized. The intensification of animal production has been progressing for many decades and centuries of time in the industrialized countries. However, man has not moved so far from his origins that it is not possible to find all levels of animal husbandry, from the most primitive to the most sophisticated so far devised, in the world of today.

This book does not set out to discuss animal management and husbandry in any detail, but it does hope to provide a basic understanding of the principles underlying the art and science of animal relationships. It is hoped that the common ground of an interest in animals will render the book of value to those who work with animals wherever they may live. The diagrams which accompany this introduction show the global pattern of animal ownership and production. While they emphasize the rather startling differences between one part of the world and another, the reader should bear in mind that this is the present situation. Many enormous pressures are shaping the structure of animal production, and these must lead to changes, in particular towards the more efficient utilization of animals in developing countries.

By far the largest proportion of the world's milk supply arises from cattle, though buffalo contribute a significant amount, and sheep and goats are also important.   Figure 1 shows that while Europe and North America produce 60% of the world's milk supply they contain only 17% of the world's cattle.   Similarly in the case of meat.   Roughly 57% of the world's meat brought into trade originates from countries which contain a third of the world's livestock populations.   These are great disparities which time will undoubtedly correct.

There are three constraints on production.   The first is the provision of adequate food and water.   Many mechanical factors exert an influence here, particularly in marginal agricultural ground and in the proximity of deserts; however these may be overcome if it proves profitable to do so.   This is the second factor—the economic restraints imposed by the distance from places where the products can be eaten or processed. The impetus of world hunger is, however, tending to make profitable management systems which would have been avoided even a few years ago.   There is therefore a pressure towards the more efficient harvesting of the products of livestock.   However, given that both these factors receive attention there is still one great restraint and one which is of the greatest interest to veterinarians and their assistants.   It is the toll that disease levies on all animal systems by producing the one wastage which can render them all sub-economic if it is not controlled.

Disease imposes a stress, and it is the veterinarian's responsibility to reduce it by any means in his power.   Nevertheless this ought not to be interpreted as a sacred duty to extend the life of every animal with which he may come into contact.   Because space on the planet is limited there is a practical necessity to terminate the lives of animals.   Within this book first aid is discussed in close conjunction with the humane destruction of animals.   The author has a belief, which he considers that he shares with many veterinarians, that man has a moral responsibility to ensure that animals should come to the end of their lives with a minimum of upset.   In other words that they should have no fear at the time of death.   This applies whether the animal has been kept by man for utilitarian or companionship reasons.

The responsibility to destroy the lives of animals need not press upon human conscience.   All animals die, and in the wild by far the greatest proportion of animals die a violent death.   In general herbivores die in the claws and teeth of a predator, and predators die of starvation or by other smaller predators, when they become too weak

WORLD PRODUCTION OF MILK

in OOO metric tonnes

I By_Species

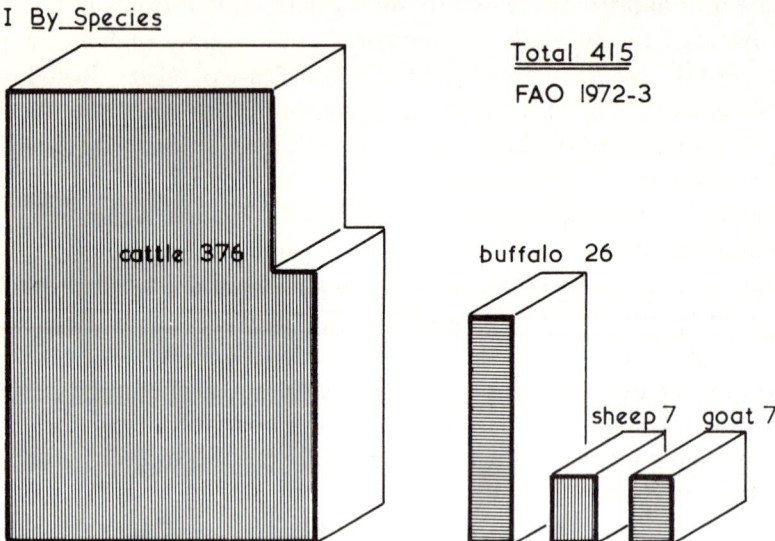

Total 415

FAO 1972-3

cattle 376

buffalo 26

sheep 7   goat 7

II By_Geographical Source

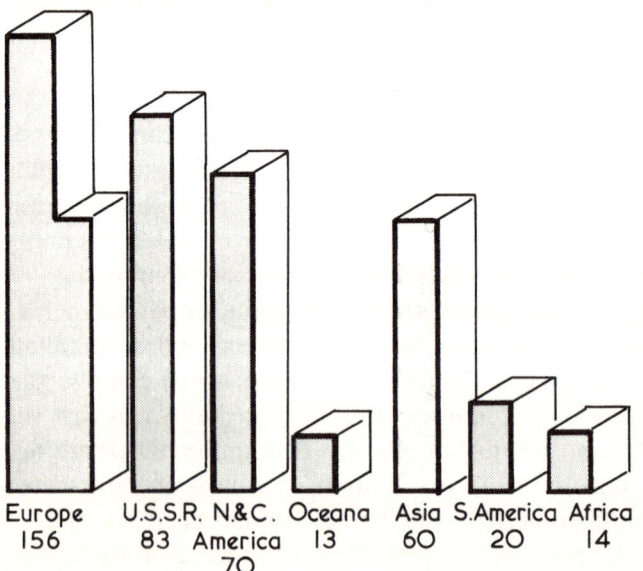

| Europe 156 | U.S.S.R. 83 | N.&C. America 70 | Oceana 13 | Asia 60 | S.America 20 | Africa 14 |

Figure 1

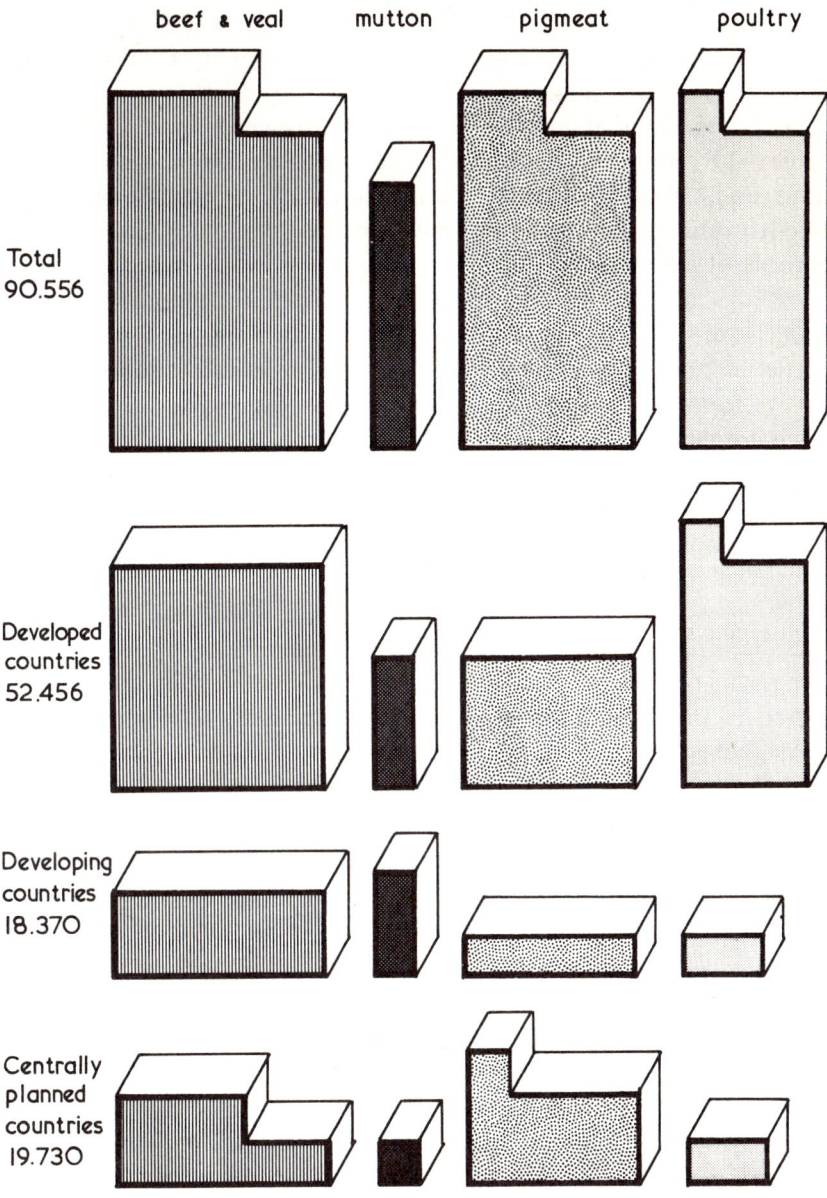

WORLD PRODUCTION OF MEAT (FAO 1972-3)
in 1000 tonnes

beef & veal   mutton   pigmeat   poultry

Total
90.556

Developed
countries
52.456

Developing
countries
18.370

Centrally
planned
countries
19.730

Figure 2

to protect themselves.   In the wild, disease may strike indiscriminately but many animals so struck down must end their lives in misery.   Those who have seen the effects of rinderpest on game animals cannot doubt this statement.   When man keeps animals for his own purposes he takes upon himself the necessity to keep them in comfort during life as well as at the point of death.

So far as can be judged a sense of contentment is more easily achieved by animals than by man.   Animals live for the day and the hour, and cannot plan for the future, nor are they capable of inductive reasoning.   There is some evidence that carnivores are more capable of learning than herbivores, but no animal is subject to introspection.   It follows therefore that animals are contented when their immediate surroundings are comfortable.   Contentment in penned cattle may be a matter of providing sufficient amounts of the right sort of food, adequate water, dry bedding and plenty of air space free from draughts.   One cannot suppose that they worry about their future, nor, if they are castrated, the absence of sexual excitement. What they have not seen they cannot regret, and it is probable that their memories are very short, and consist mainly of remembered danger or stress.

The message is therefore that restriction of itself is not harmful, provided that in planning that restriction one takes into account the behaviour pattern of the species.   Animals are not human beings in fur coats, but this fact only increases the necessity to relieve them of avoidable stress.   On many occasions destruction without pain is less stressful than prolonged unsuccessful treatment.

Because the presence of disease is so stressful it is important that its nature should be diagnosed as soon as possible.   A section of this book has therefore been devoted to the nature of disease and the methods available for its diagnosis.   Of equal importance is the understanding of health; a healthy animal is one which behaves normally so some knowledge of the behaviour patterns of each species is essential.   No matter what stage one has reached in the study of animals, it is of value to know the limits of treatment and the relative importance of specific disease. This too is covered in general principle.

Lastly it is hoped that the book will provide a means of reference once general instruction is complete and useful tables and a glossary have been supplied.

The object of this book is to stimulate interest.   It can only be a first step in studying veterinary science, but the more one thinks about animals the more deeply one becomes involved.   This book will have served its purpose if it helps people to understand animals, and perhaps through that understanding to sympathize with the problems of others with similar interests in all parts of the world.

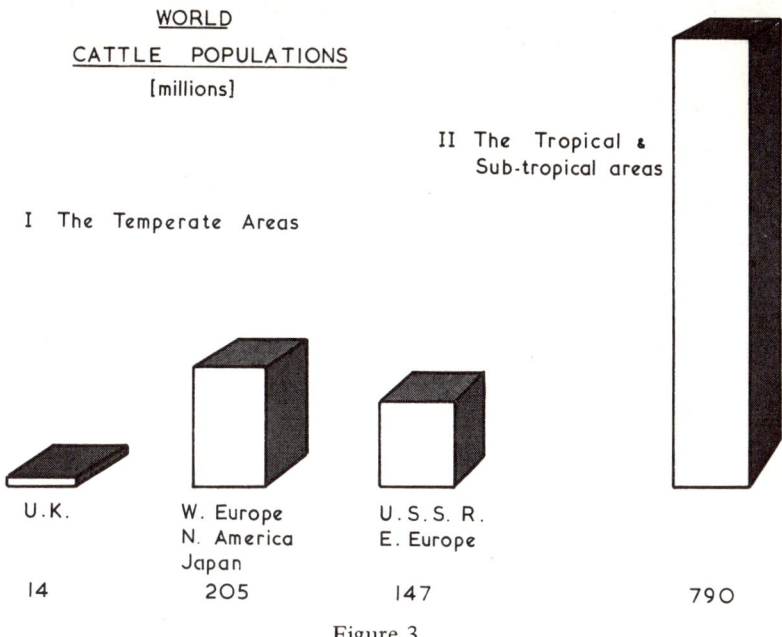

WORLD

CATTLE   POPULATIONS

[millions]

II   The   Tropical &
Sub-tropical areas

I   The   Temperate   Areas

U.K.

W. Europe
N. America
Japan

U.S.S.R.
E. Europe

14

205

147

790

Figure 3

It is hoped that the reader will be left with the following thoughts in respect of his attitude to animals.

(1) Man's civilization has been possible because of his association with animals.

(2) Man is still dependent on animals for the food they provide, particularly in the form of readily available protein.

(3) Animal protein is probably in over-supply in some parts of the world, but more important, it is in under-supply in many other parts.

(4) In many countries animals still offer the most economical form of transport and traction.

(5) The comfort of animal companionship should not be under-estimated nor scorned.   Companion animals may be a necessity for human beings living in crowded communities.

- (6) Healthy animals are desirable from every respect, and disease control offers a continuing and rewarding interest.

(7) It is irresponsible not to tie animal disease control with the utilization of the animals which have survived by its practice.   Animal population control is as important as human population control, and much easier to achieve.

(8) There is little to indicate that man will be able to dispense with animals in the foreseeable future.   He has therefore to control disease in animals as a part of his own protection against infection.

Section I

Anatomy and Physiology

THE STRUCTURE AND FUNCTION OF THE BODY

The body is formed of millions of cells, each one a separate form of life, independent in that it is capable of taking in food and building substances, translating them into energy, and excreting the waste products that result, but interdependent on the other cells for the means of existence. Each cell is supported physically by its neighbours, and together they contribute to the efficiency of the organ in which they are found.

Each organ performs one or more specialized functions which enable the body to survive. For instance the body tissues and other organs are covered either by skin, or, in the case of the surfaces of the intestinal tract, the reproductive tract, and the sense organs, by mucous membranes. This covering is a vital protective mechanism against many hazards of the outside world; it is only when this covering has been destroyed or successfully invaded that damage and disease takes place. To perform this protective function the skin is supplied with highly specialized cells which have developed the capacity to secrete a leathery covering, known as *keratin*, or to produce hair or fur.

The specialized cells in every organ have to be supported by stiffening material or connective tissue. Some organs have more of this material than others, but it is the connective tissue that supports the characteristic shape of the various organs, and which keeps them remarkably similar in shape within the species of animal. It is also

necessary that the organ should be supplied with food substances
and that the means should be available to carry away waste products.
This function is supplied by the blood.   Cells are composed largely
of water surrounded by a membrane, and the water molecules together
with the molecules of other substances carried in solution or suspension
move readily to and fro through this covering.   It is the constant flow
of blood to and from the organ which maintains the correct balance
of molecules to enable the cells to function correctly.   The blood is
carried in blood vessels which form a maze of tiny tubes or capillaries
within the organ they serve.   Each one of these capillaries is made up
of stretched out and flattened cells which form the capillary walls.
The blood also carries cells; the red ones give it its characteristic red
colour, and the white or colourless cells are concerned with protection
against disease.   White cells are mobile and work their way into and
out of capillaries by edging their way between the lining cells.

Each organ receives messages; some of them are transmitted to it
by chemicals contained in the blood but others are relayed perhaps
more rapidly along the nerves by electrical impulse.   Each nerve is
made up of the very elongated process of nerve cells which link up
with other nerve cell processes at nerve junctions.   The effect is to
produce rapid transmission of messages to all parts of the body, so
stimulating the actions that are needed if the animal is to survive.

There is another liquid which bathes the organs.   This is lymphatic
fluid or *lymph* and it is moved around the body by means of the
lymphatic vessels.   The lymphatic vessels are interrupted at intervals
by small or large accumulations of tissue which are found in organs
or on the course of the vessels.   These are the lymph glands, each of
which contains numerous small white cells known as *lymphocytes*,
and which act as filters of the fluid which passes through them.
During the course of many diseases tissue debris forms in the organs
as a result of the constant battle waged by white cells which try to
engulf the invading organisms.   This debris composed of dead cells,
and perhaps organisms, is strained out of the lymph by the lymph
glands.   Often this produces an inflammatory response in the gland,
which swells as the tissues continue to combat the infection by
mobilizing many more white cells.   Enlarged lymph glands are a
feature of many diseases.

Each organ is seen to consist of many types of cells.   Some types
are found in all parts of the body, either because they are carried

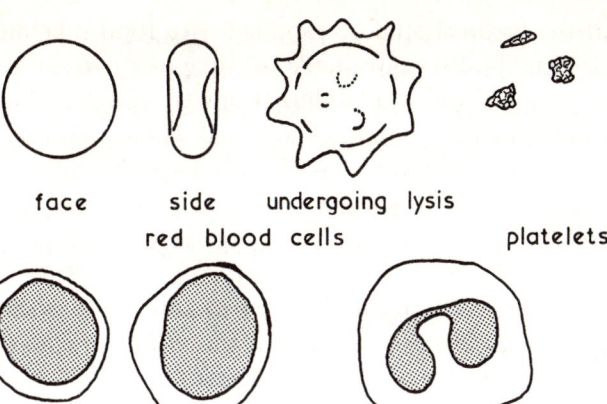

face   side   undergoing lysis

red blood cells   platelets

lymphocytes   white blood cell

CELLULAR CONSTITUENTS OF BLOOD

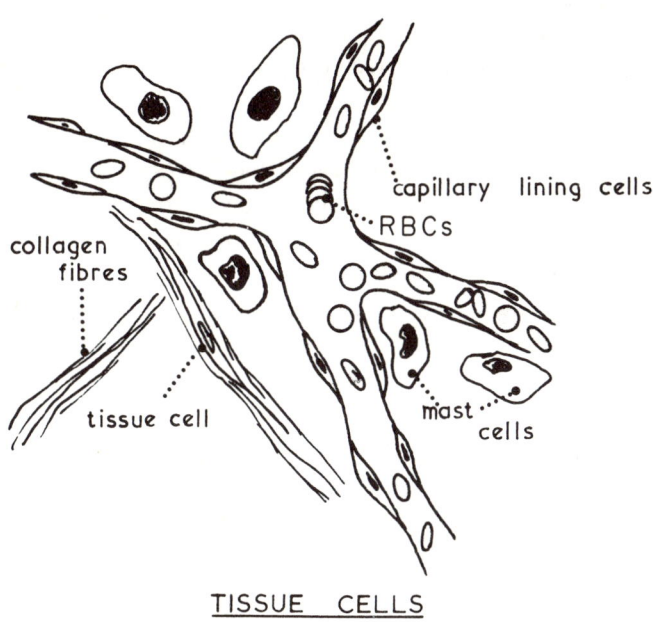

capillary   lining cells

RBCs

collagen
fibres

tissue cell

mast
cells

TISSUE CELLS

Figure 4

there by the blood stream, or because they are tissue cells common
to all body systems.   An example of the former type of cell are
those which form components of the blood, and of the latter, cells
which form part of the walls of capillaries as well as cells involved in

the building structure of tissues.   These are tissue cells which are concerned with the production of fibres known as *collagen* fibres. Besides these commonly found cells each organ contains specialized cells.   Their individual function, and to some extent the form in which they are found, determines their location.   For instance, liver cells are only found in liver, because in that site they are able to convert products brought to them in the blood stream into substances which the animal can use.

The organs combine together to form a number of specialized systems which are described in some detail in the following pages. All these systems are dependent one on the other; none of them may work or exert its effect in isolation, if the animal is to adapt satisfactorily to its surroundings.   The skeletal system provides the hard bony structure from which the parts of the body are suspended, and the muscular system provides the work mechanism of movement. Muscular movement is achieved by rhythmic contraction and relaxation.   The circulatory system carries the chemical messengers and food substances around the body.   The digestive system enables food in crude form to be taken into and stored within the body, so that it can be broken down into a form in which it can be absorbed for transport in the circulatory system.   The respiratory system allows the assimilation of oxygen and the excretion of excess water and of carbon dioxide.   The excretory system disposes of waste products, and the central nervous system organizes the body's responses.   The reproductive system enables the body to perpetuate the species and the endocrine system provides chemical messengers to regulate body functions.

Reproduction is given the utmost priority by healthy, sexually intact, mature animals.   The urge to reproduce is only second to that of individual survival.   This being so it is not surprising that the act of reproduction should have such profound effects on many organs and should provide the greatest hazard to the life of the female.

The impact of this introduction will be achieved if the reader comes to appreciate the following points:

(1) The smallest unit in the body is the cell.   Each cell is self-reliant to the point of survival and reproduction but is supported by its neighbours and serviced by body fluids.

(2) Each organ is composed of specialist cells, connective tissue cells, capillary wall cells, blood cells and lymph cells or lymphocytes

(-cyte means cell, so cells are given a name ending in cyte).

(3) Each organ has a specialized function to perform within a body system.

(4) While the systems are described separately they are in reality all inter-dependent. Any factor which radically affects one system will affect others. In other words an injury or the effect of a disease is rarely confined to one organ.

(5) An animal's first objective is to survive, its second, sometimes at the hazard of the first, is to reproduce itself.

THE SKELETAL SYSTEM

The skeleton is composed of a number of bones connected to each other by joints, and acting as a framework for the soft tissues and organs of the body. Essentially it is a system of levers, and so affords a means of locomotion.

Parts of the skeleton

The skeleton is divisible into two main parts: (1) the axial skeleton, and (2) the skeleton of the limbs and girdles. The former occupies the main axis of the body and consists of the skull and the vertebral column together with the ribs. The remainder of the skeleton consists of the fore and hind limbs together with the bones to which they are attached.

The skull

The skull consists of a number of bones which, joined together, form the head. The upper part, called the *cranium*, encloses and protects the brain. The lower part is called the *mandible* or lower jaw. The hole, or *foramen*, in the centre carries the spinal cord to the brain. The cranium also carries the nasal passages, the orbits where the eyes are placed and contains the hearing system.

The spine or vertebral column

The spine or vertebral column is a series of bones which run from the head to the end of the tail. Each of the bones of the spine is called a *vertebra*. Each vertebra has a foramen at its centre through which the spinal cord passes.

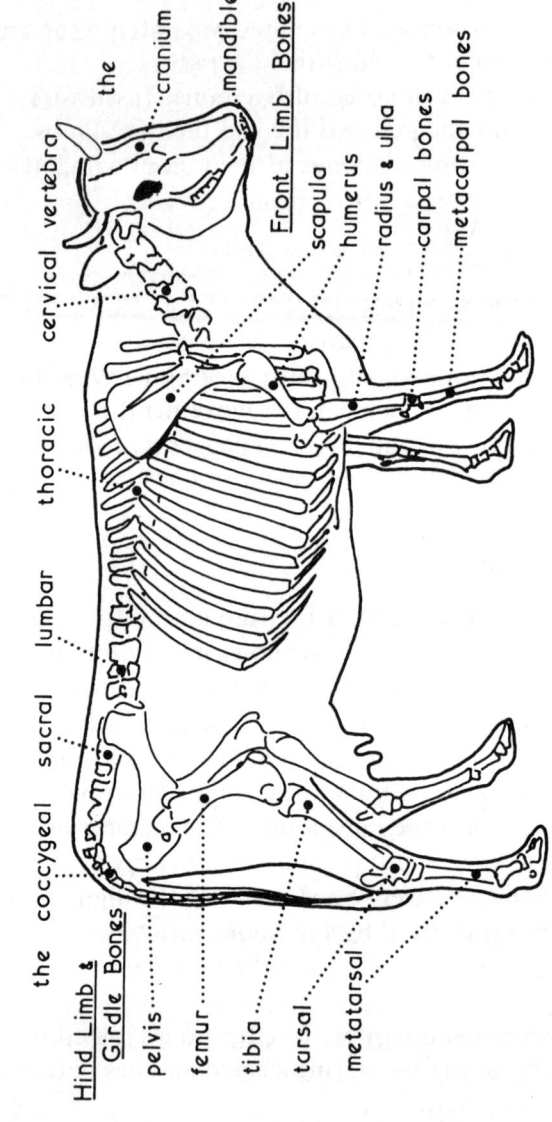

THE SKELETON OF THE COW

The Axial Skeleton

the   coccygeal   sacral   lumbar   thoracic   cervical vertebra   the   cranium &   mandible

Front Limb Bones

scapula
humerus
radius & ulna
carpal bones
metacarpal bones

Hind Limb &
Girdle Bones

pelvis
femur
tibia
tarsal
metatarsal

Figure 5

The spine is divided into five groups of vertebra:

Cervical vertebrae or neck bones, of which there are seven.

Thoracic vertebrae or chest bones to which are attached the ribs, and of which there are thirteen.

Lumbar vertebrae of which there are six.

Sacrum, which is composed of five bones fused together to form a rigid support for the pelvic girdle and the hind limbs.

Coccygeal vertebrae or bones of the tail, of which there are eighteen to twenty.

The chest or thorax

The chest or thorax is made up of the ribs and the breastbone.   There are thirteen pairs of ribs in cattle.   They extend from the vertebral column to the breastbone and form a cage enclosing the thorax. They are of great importance in the movements responsible for the filling and emptying of the lungs.   The *sternum* or breastbone makes the floor of the thoracic cavity or chest, and is formed of segments of bone and cartilage.

The fore limb

The *scapula* is the first bone of the fore limb.   It is a triangular-shaped flat bone which is attached to the body mainly by muscles.   The *humerus* is the next bone.   With the scapula, it forms the shoulder joint.   The lower end of the humerus forms the elbow joint with the *radius* and *ulna* which are joined together side by side.   Next come the *carpal bones*, six in number, four in the top row and two in the bottom.   These form the knee joint.   The *metacarpal* is the long bone below the knee and it is followed by two sets of three short bones called the *phalanges* which make up the digits or toes.   The lowest phalange is covered by the hoof.

The pelvis

The pelvis consists of a number of large bones joined together.   It is the largest bone in the body, ring-shaped and lies between the lumbar vertebrae and the sacrum.

The hind limb

On each side of the pelvis is a hollow cup called the *acetabulum* into which fits the top of the *femur* or first bone of the hind limb forming the hip joint.   The femur is a long strong bone which is joined at its lower end to the *tibia* to form the stifle joint in the front of which is also included the *patella* or knee-cap.   At the lower end of the tibia come the tarsal bones, five in number.   With the top end of the *metatarsal* they form the hock joint.   The metatarsal is a long bone below which are the two sets of three phalanges as in the fore limb.

SURFACE   POINT   RECOGNITION

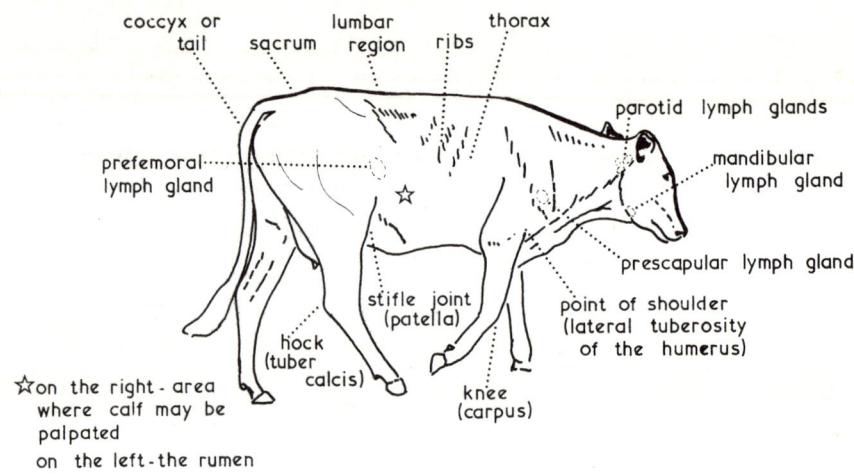

Figure 6

A joint

A joint is the meeting of two or more bones, e.g. the elbow joint where the humerus, radius and ulna meet, allowing the fore limb to be bent at that place.

A ligament

A ligament is a strong band of tissue which ties two bones together.

Movement of the body

Joints allow the skeleton to be flexible and, by the action of the muscles and tendons, enable the various parts of the body to be moved at will.

The joint is completely enclosed in the joint capsule attached to the two bones.   It consists of an outer, fibrous layer and an internal layer, the synovial membrane, which produces *synovial fluid* to lubricate the movements of the joint.   The two bones are held together at various points by *ligaments* which are the thickest parts of the joint capsule fibrous layer.

Tendons are dense, fibrous, slightly elastic cords that attach the ends of muscles to the bones, or other structures upon which the

<u>MUSCLES & TENDONS</u>   <u>JOINTS</u>

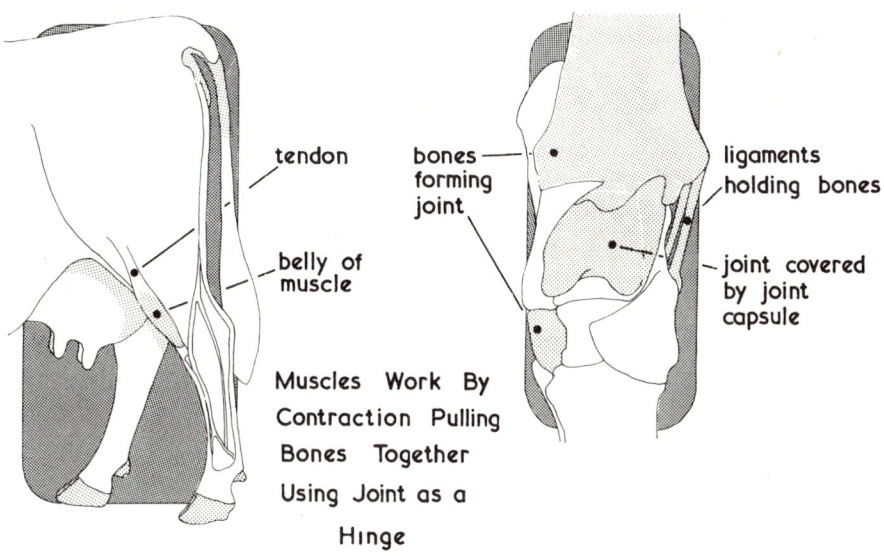

Figure 7

muscles act when they contract.   They are white in colour.   They may also be called *sinews*.   They are carried in sheaths lined with a lubricating membrane similar to that found in joint cavities so that they slide easily.   Muscles work by contraction.   When a muscle contracts the attached tendon is pulled up and the bone to which it is attached at its lower end is moved accordingly.   By a succession of muscles acting on bones through the tendons, the animal is able to walk, run, lie down, etc.

The teeth of animals

Teeth have become considerably modified in different species of animals in order that they may be adapted to the type of food that is eaten. The requirement for herbivorous animals is that they should be able to cut grass and other herbage off close to the ground. Therefore in vegetarian animals, the incisors or front teeth are very well developed as cutting instruments. Once the grass is in the mouth, it must be crushed, and in herbivorous animals the large molars or back teeth have developed into table-like, flat upper surfaces. These can grind the food between the upper and lower jaws, and make it more suitable for the action of enzymes which seek to break it up into substances which can be absorbed by the digestive tract.

In the carnivorous animals, that is those which eat flesh and must therefore be able to seize and hold prey, as well as to eat tough food substances, different modifications are needed. Their teeth look completely different from those of herbivores. The teeth which lie between the incisors and molars are known as the canine teeth and are long and strong in animals like dogs and cats. In addition, one molar on each side of each jaw is developed into a strong sharp edge which can be used to cut away the meat. These are known as the *carnassials*.

The pig possesses the full complement of teeth; on each side of each jaw are three incisors, one canine, four premolars and three molars. It is an omnivore, that is it will eat any sort of food presented to it; perhaps the original mammal from which all others have developed looked something like a small pig.

The rabbit and the rat have greatly enlarged incisors since they are adapted to chewing roots and bark as well as grass. The incisors of a rodent grow continuously and they are worn down against each other during life.

In all mammals the young animal first grows a set of milk or deciduous teeth. These are gradually replaced by the permanent teeth at a later stage in life. Normally it is the incisors, the canines, and the first three molars in each side of each jaw which are grown as milk teeth. The hind molars erupt by themselves as the jaw grows to accommodate them.

The ageing of animals by their teeth

Teeth grow slowly and while the bodies of meat animals may grow quite rapidly, their age may be detected by their teeth. Only the bottom jaw of cattle carries incisors. The young calf is born with four temporary incisors which are replaced from the middle outwards.   The first pair of replacements arrives at $1\frac{1}{2}$–2 years of age; the others are replaced at roughly six monthly intervals until all the

THE TEETH OF ANIMALS

Pig's jaw with comparisons

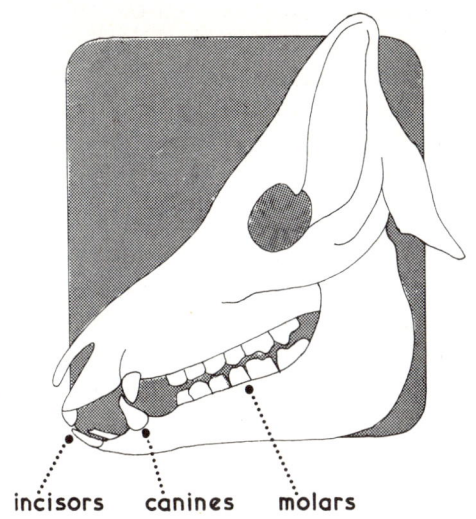

incisors   canines   molars

Cattle & Sheep	no incisors upper jaw
Dogs & Cats	modified canines & molars
Horses	big gap between modified strong incisors & molars
Rodents	modified incisors

Figure 8

permanent incisors are present at four years of age.   In Europe, many beef animals are slaughtered just at the time that the first pair of incisors is erupting.

It has become traditional to age horses by their teeth.   The same principles apply as in cattle but because horses live longer, it is necessary to go further than merely counting permanent incisors.   Most estimates of age are carried out as the horse ages and progressively

wears down the tooth enamel, exposing first the dentine and then
the tooth cavity in very old animals.   It must be apparent however
that ageing from the teeth in animals in excess of ten years cannot be
very precise, because teeth wear at different rates between individuals.
However, the eruption times of the permanent incisors are fairly
standard, and most horses have a full mouth at five years of age.
Confusion can arise in comparing a one-year-old animal (a yearling)
with a five-year-old in that each has a full mouth of incisors but the
former are temporary and the latter permanent.

The charts give the complement of teeth and the age in respect of
eruption and wear for the domestic animals.

Other signs of ageing in animals

In horses and cattle, hollows appear around the eyes as the orbital fat
becomes decreased in amount.   White hairs appear, particularly at the
muzzle, and in the horse the lips tend to sag.   The muscles of the
abdomen also lose their tension and the belly appears more rounded.

The horns in cattle provide another means of ageing; one ring
equals one year of life; add 2 to give the estimated age.   Similarly,
the hooves of both animals get a worn look and are not as smooth as
in the young animal.   There are exceptions to every rule but the
following are the main signs of age in animals:

Cows: The cow's udder and feet bear the strain of a long life, the
one become more pendulous and the hooves longer and ridged.   In
horned animals the horns become long with many rings.

Horses: It is teeth and legs of a horse which carry the strain,
in particular the legs, and it is rare indeed for the limbs of a ten-year-
old horse to be without blemish.   The teeth are usually examined
but cannot be expected to pinpoint the age precisely in aged animals.

Dogs: In heavy dogs the signs are more apparent than in light ones;
they include greying of the muzzle and staining and wear of the
canine and carnassial teeth.   An old dog can be considerably helped
by tooth care.

Cats: Cats are difficult to age and, perhaps because they are light
in weight, usually carry their age well.   The teeth usually give away
the age in an old animal and here again care in cleaning the teeth can
improve an old cat's well-being.

DENTAL FORMULAE OF ANIMALS

	Incisors	Canines	Molars
Teeth of Horses			
Top jaws	6	2	12–14
Bottom jaws	6	2	12–14

Note: At one year all temporary incisors in wear. At $4\frac{1}{2}$–5 years all permanent incisors in wear.

	Incisors	Canines	Molars
Teeth of Cattle			
Top jaws	0	0	12
Bottom jaws	8	0	12

Note: Cattle with central permanent incisors cut should be regarded as over 1 year 6 months of age. Cattle with central permanent incisors fully up–1 year 9 months. Cattle with all permanent incisors up are regarded as being over 3 years of age.

	Incisors	Canines	Molars
Teeth of Sheep			
Top jaws	0	0	12
Bottom jaws	8	0	12

Note: First pair of permanent incisors appear at 1 year to 1 year 3 months. All permanent teeth are present at 3 years of age.

	Incisors	Canines	Molars
Teeth of Pigs			
Top jaws	6	2	14
Bottom jaws	6	2	14

	Incisors	Canines	Molars
Teeth of Dogs			
Top jaws	6	2	12
Bottom jaws	6	2	12

Note: Puppies are born without teeth, the temporary teeth gradually appear and the permanent canines are usually present by 7 months of age.

THE MUSCULAR SYSTEM

In general animal cells have two properties or abilities; they may contract or they may secrete, and they may specialize in either function. Muscle tissue, the substance commonly recognized as meat, is composed of long cells which have the ability to contract. All movement by animals is therefore the result of contraction and subsequent relaxation of muscle cells.

Voluntary muscles

There are some muscle movements which have to be in the constant control of the animal; these are regarded as being voluntary because they power the muscles connected to parts of the skeleton.   As has been shown, the skeleton itself is hinged together at the joints in such a way that it may be moved in any way that the joint allows. By a wonderful system of muscle connection, and control of contraction, all the complex movements of the animal become possible.

It follows that each muscle has to be isolated or separated from its fellows, and this is done by means of a muscle sheath of connective tissue, which has the additional important function of friction-free movement over the muscles lying around it.   It is connected through a tendon at one end of the muscle to a prominence or attachment on a bone and similarly at the other end to another bone across the joint, and again through a tendon.   It follows that each voluntary muscle may be dissected out from its fellows and seen in its entirety.

Muscles are in active movement for long periods of time and require considerable amounts of energy.   This is supplied to them by arteries which divide down into small capillaries, giving the muscle tissue a high volume of blood supply.   The burning of energy produces waste materials and these are carried away in the veins.   The action of muscles is very carefully organized by the brain; many of the movements, while voluntary in the sense that the brain has control over the function, are to some extent automatic because brain links have been formed by practice which causes response to certain stimuli without prolonged thought.   These are known as *reflex actions*.   A simple analogy is provided by the motor car; the driver does not have to think so that the right piston shall fire in sequence; once he has decided to start the engine, it turns over by automatic response.   This leaves the driver or the 'brain' of the car free to decide where to go and at what speed to travel.

The importance and complexity of action of voluntary muscles may be gained from the facts that over 700 separate muscles are to be found in the body and that muscles account for 30% of the dead weight of an ox carcase.

Involuntary muscles

A little thought will show that it is not practical to have voluntary muscular control over certain body functions.   The sort of actions which spring immediately to mind are those which push food along the intestine, or which power the heart.   Equally certain functions of

TYPES OF MUSCLE CELL

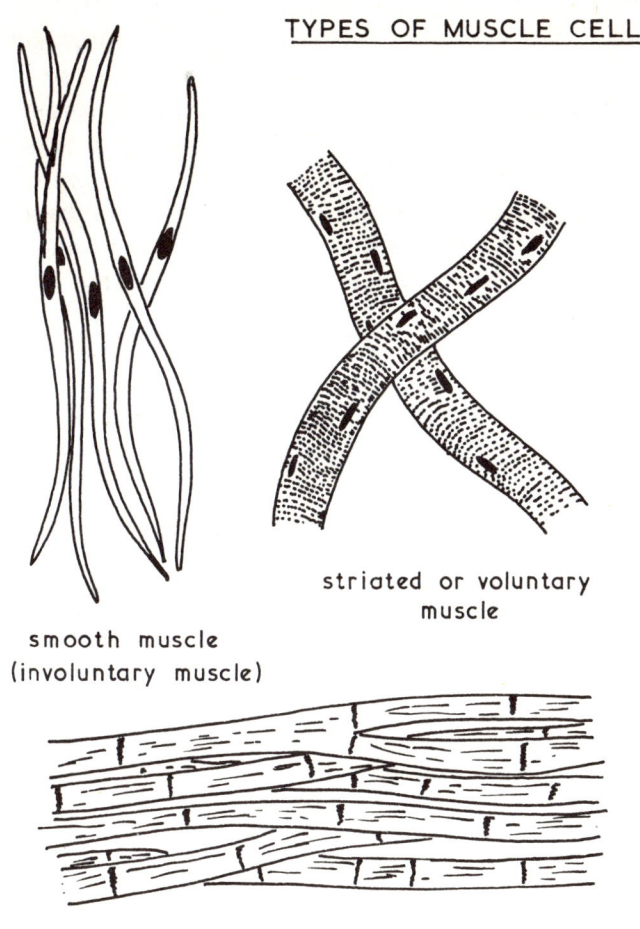

striated or voluntary
muscle

smooth muscle
(involuntary muscle)

heart muscle

Figure 9

muscle are halfway between voluntary and involuntary movements, in that, while the action to relax or contract is under conscious thought in part, the degree of relaxation or contraction cannot be controlled.   These are the muscles which control exit and entry of fluid in hollow organs.

The big difference between voluntary and involuntary muscles is that in the latter instance the muscles do not have defined form and they are frequently found in conjunction with other types of cells. The movement of food along the intestine is by a process known as *peristalsis.* This is a rhythmic contraction of the intestinal wall accomplished by involuntary muscles contained within its tissue. The movement appears to be in response to physical factors such as distention by the passage of food or water, and is quite independent of conscious thought, although the sequence of the rhythmic contractions is under the control of nerves low down in the vertebral column. Coordinated intestinal movements may be seen in the recently dead animal but these become incoordinated as the nerve cells die progressively along the spinal cord.

Most hollow organs contain great quantities of involuntary muscle fibres which by their contraction reduce the capacity of the organ. The bladder is a typical case in point. Contraction of the wall enables the organ to force urine out down the ureter so that it is voided outside the body.

This brings into prominence the type of action of involuntary muscles already referred to, in which the action is in some degree conscious, in that it is started by a message from the brain. These are the *sphincter* muscles which by contraction close the exit from a vessel. Examples are found at the anus, at the point where the stomach leads into the intestine, and at the exit to the bladder.

The heart muscle is a very special case and will be considered under the circulatory system.

THE CIRCULATORY SYSTEM

The main requirement for the continuation of life is that tissues and organs should be supplied with fuel: in essence this is the transport of oxygen from the lungs, and the movement of food substances from the intestine through the liver. The oxygenation or burning of that fuel involves the production of waste products, and these too must be moved away before they can cause damage to the cells. These functions are maintained by the circulatory fluid, or blood, which is carried within the closed circulatory system.

The composition of the blood

All animals originated in the sea.   It is thought that when single-celled animals like the *amoeba* developed into multicellular organisms, and when later they adopted the increased complexity of a body cavity, they trapped within themselves a little of the sea in which they had developed.   Because this early sea, which covered the greater part of the globe, had fewer minerals dissolved in it than is now the case, mammalian body fluids are far less salty than the sea with which we are now familiar.

Whatever the origin of body fluid, the basic constituent of blood is water in which are dissolved a number of electrolytes, minerals and organic compounds.   The degree of alkalinity or acidity of this fluid is of the greatest importance to the survival of the animal, because the body processes have evolved to function at a constant pH value.   The blood therefore contains considerable 'buffering' powers to enable it to maintain these levels while carrying in circulation all the substances required to support *metabolism*.   The methods employed to do this are complex; suffice it to say here that an important function of the blood is to maintain the fluid surrounding tissue cells at a constant chemical level.

The blood carries oxygen to the tissues and carries away carbon dioxide, in addition to other substances.   All energy depends ultimately on chemical action in the presence of oxygen to produce energy, while the maintenance of the correct pH depends on the elimination of carbon dioxide which causes acidity.   It is clear that the blood could not produce the quantity of oxygen required by heavy muscular effort merely by transporting it in solution.

The oxygen is conveyed by attachment to a complex protein molecule known as *haemoglobin*, which is contained within the red blood cells, or RBCs.   The attachment of oxygen to haemoglobin turns it scarlet in colour; this red pigment gives the blood in the arteries such a characteristic appearance.   When the oxygen is released in the tissues the red blood cells revert to their natural bluish colour, so venous blood is blue.

It has been said that haemoglobin is the most important chemical in the body since it makes possible the act of respiration.   Multicellular animals could not have developed without it since otherwise they would be dependant for existence on oxygen dissolved in water.   It follows therefore that any illness or poison which prevents the blood from carrying oxygen will result immediately in serious consequences for the affected animal. Certain blood parasites destroy the RBCs, so reducing the amount of oxygen which can be transported. Monoxide poisoning results in the fixing of the haemoglobin by a tight combination with oxygen which cannot therefore be released in the tissues. Again this results in oxygen starvation or *anoxia.*

SCHEMATIC REPRESENTATION OF THE BLOOD CIRCULATION

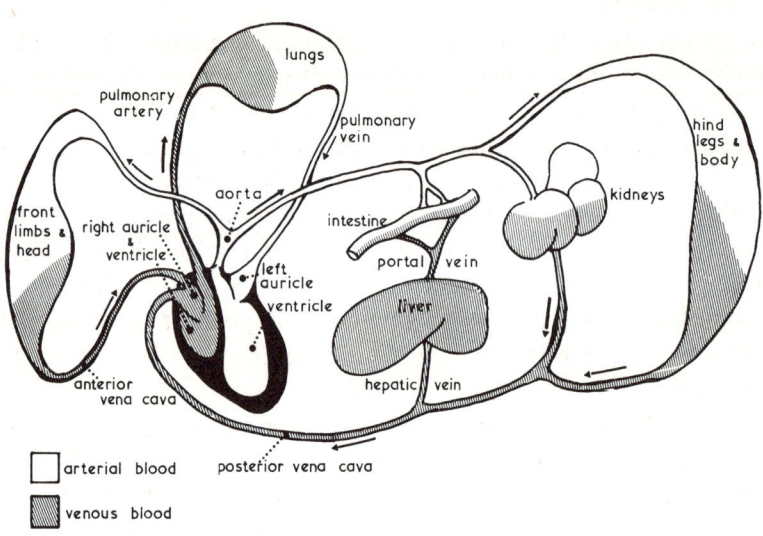

Figure 10

In addition to the RBCs a number of other types of cell are carried in the blood. There are several varieties of white blood cell; these have a nucleus and an irregular outline, and their main task is the envelopment within their cytoplasm of particles invading the body. They may be thought of as scavengers which accumulate where infection has gained entry, and which try to eliminate the cause of injury. Another important cellular-type constituent of blood is the platelet, which is present in large quantities and which has an important part in clotting.

The clotting of blood

There are three stages to the clotting of blood. When blood flow is stopped by a wound the platelets produce a substance which combines with protein from the damaged tissue to produce a substance known as *thrombin*. Thrombin combines with a protein known as *fibrinogen*, which is present in normal blood plasma, to form a series of threads of *fibrin*. The network of threads so formed holds up the cellular constituents of the blood, first producing a deep red clot because of the large numbers of RBCs. This becomes yellow in colour as the fibres contract forcing out the *serum* (plasma without clotting compounds) and leaving behind numerous white cells which start the process of healing.

The heart and the circulation

The heart is a muscular organ which by regular controlled contraction of its four component chambers forces blood around the body. The well-known heart beat is produced by the closing of the valves which separate the chambers one from the other, and which have the function of preventing back flow of blood. With care it is possible to recognize the part that each valve contributes to the heart sound and, in the abnormal heart, to diagnose faults in any particular valve.

There are two types of chamber in the heart. The two *auricles* or entrance chambers are thin walled, and store the blood until the valves open to allow it to enter the muscular *ventricles*. The ventricles lead into *arteries* which are vessels with strong elastic walls. The left ventricle opens into the aorta, which is also guarded by valves, and this main artery divides and subdivides to provide a closed route for the blood entering the tissues. Within the tissues and organs the arterioles (or smallest arteries) divide into numerous capillaries. Many of these capillaries remain closed while the animal is at rest and requiring little oxygen, but they can open to enrich the supply in case of need. The capillaries open into the small veins which gradually converge until they enter the large venous trunks which return the blood to the heart. One of the most important veins in the body is the one which collects the blood from the intestine and feeds it through the liver on its way to the heart. In the liver food substances are filtered out and processed, to be added eventually to the venous blood in a form in which they can be used by body cells.

The route that blood takes in the circulation is shown in the diagram, and it is only necessary here to point out certain factors. It will be clear that the pulmonary artery carries blue de-oxygenated blood to the lungs, and that the pulmonary veins carry red oxygenated blood from the lungs to the heart. By increasing the heart rate it is

THE CIRCULATION OF THE
BLOOD

(illustrated on the heart of an Ox)

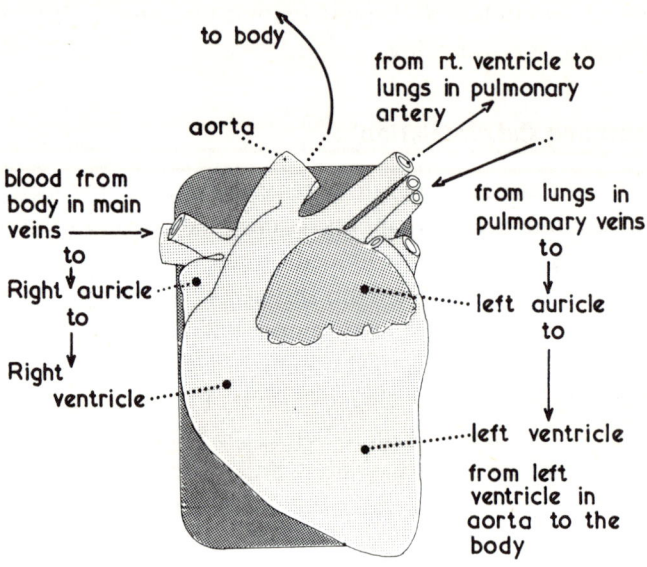

to body

from rt. ventricle to lungs in pulmonary artery

aorta

blood from body in main veins ———→ to Right ▼ auricle to Right ▼ ventricle

from lungs in pulmonary veins to left auricle to left ventricle

from left ventricle in aorta to the body

Red oxygenated blood in pulmonary veins and in left auricle and ventricle, and main arteries.

Blue de-oxygenated blood in main veins and in right auricle & ventricle.

Figure 11

possible to increase the flow of blood.   However, it would not be efficient to increase the blood flow to all tissues if the need was not universally apparent.   There is therefore both chemical and involuntary nervous control over the degree to which the capillaries may be opened by the force of the circulation.   Equally there are organs such as the brain which must receive the best circulation possible, since brain cells require a high concentration of oxygen with which to perform their function.

The pool of blood that can be held within the capillaries should they all dilate at once is very considerable. In shock, which is the result of extreme stress, retention occurs and the animal becomes noticeably pale. Note that there need be no gross damage to blood vessels for this to occur, merely an opening of too many terminal tissue vessels all at once. This type of blood stasis can be a cause of death unless urgent remedial measures are taken.

The circulatory system and the health of the animal

At rest the heart maintains a regular beat which produces pressure pulses in the arteries corresponding to the forcing of the blood around the system. Because the walls of the arteries are elastic in nature they respond to the increased amount of blood forced into them by expanding. It is this wave of pressure moving along the vessels like a ripple, which can be detected in the live animal by gently trapping a limb artery against a bone with the fingers. With practice, a considerable amount of information about the health of the animal can be deduced from experience of variations in the pulse rate.

Two major functions influence pulse rate; firstly the forceful contraction of the heart, and secondly the amount of blood that the heart is able to push around the system. Any injury or disease which restricts the beat of the heart will affect the pulse rate, and when there has been extensive haemorrhage or bleeding there will be insufficient blood in the system to provide a firm beat. As explained it is not only bleeding which reduces the blood available to the heart. In 'shock' many of the capillaries dilate at the same time, and this sudden loss of blood to the tissues severely reduces the available blood supply in circulation, and hence produces a weak pulse. Pulse rates vary between animal species and are faster in young animals than in adults.

It will also be apparent that the composition of the blood is of importance to the maintenance of health. The pulse rate will supply a rough guide to the amount of fluid in circulation at any one time, but it is no indication of its consistency.

Water is the main constituent of the blood and has some valuable physical properties. It is a good transporter of chemicals, it is extremely stable, is a good conductor of heat, and is incompressible. Without water, life is impossible, and the more water is restricted the

more difficult it is for animals to survive, let alone grow and reproduce.
The circulatory mechanism and the consistency of the blood is maintained in times of water shortage by drawing it out of the tissues.
The very thirsty animal has the appearance of having shrunk in upon
itself. Finally in the last stages of thirst circulation becomes impossible and the animal dies.

Blood has therefore the properties of water, and makes those
properties available to the body. It maintains the body temperature,
it excretes excess fluid, and draws upon the body's water resources in
times of need. Blood transports oxygen, carbon dioxide, food substances, hormones and waste products and, last but by no means least,
it provides the body with its means of combating disease.

The lymphatic system

The arterial, capillary and venous system is only one way in which
fluids circulate through body tissues. It is a closed system from which
substances move out and in either by diffusion and osmosis or, in the
case of white blood cells, by active movement. However it has already been mentioned that tissues are bathed in lymph which is in
direct contact with cells. There is an obvious need for a watery solution in close contact with the intimate structure of organs. Metabolism or the chemical organization of body function is only possible
by means of the exchange of biological substances in water. Lymph
is a liquid with a close affinity to plasma but rendered cloudy by the
large numbers of lymphocytes that it contains.

The function of lymph glands as filters of lymph has already been
explained. There are certain chronic disease conditions which may
be detected by the presence of significant lesions in the lymph glands.
The most obvious of these is tuberculosis. Tubercles are formed by
the large white cells, known as *macrophages*, enveloping the tubercle
bacillus (*Mycobacterium tuberculosis* in the case of man) and travelling with the organism contained in the protoplasm to the lymph
glands. Here the large cells are retained by the fibrous nature of the
gland. It is a feature of tuberculosis that animals susceptible to the
disease are unable to destroy the bacteria within the enveloping cells.
Macrophages absorb the bacilli which are thus protected from circulating antibody. The end result is a growing *necrotic* lesion in the
lymph gland.

LYMPH NODES IN BOVINE CARCASE

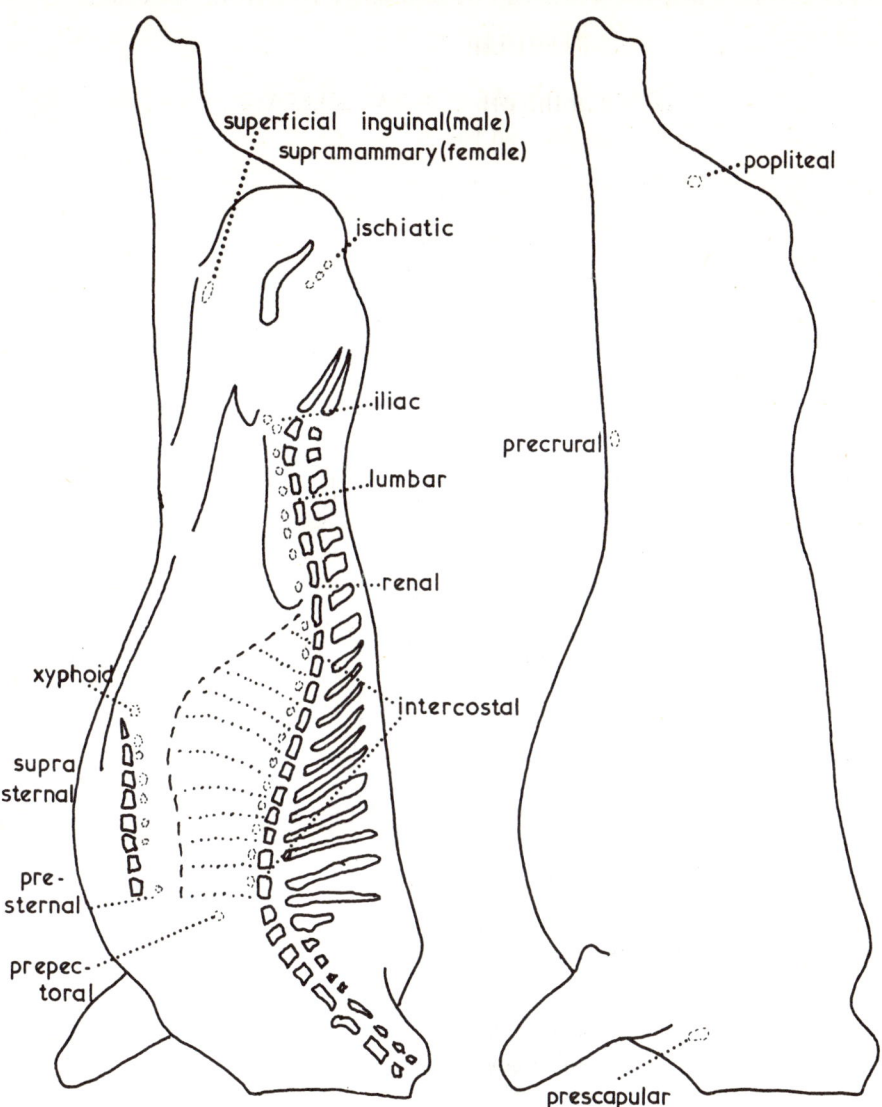

Figure 12

One necessary function of meat inspection is to open the lymph glands of animals slaughtered for food to see if they contain such evidence of infection.   The diagrams illustrate the places where the most prominent carcase lymphatics are to be found.   There are however lymph glands in the other organs which must also be examined before a whole carcase can be said to be free from infection.

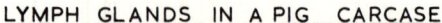

LYMPH GLANDS IN A PIG CARCASE

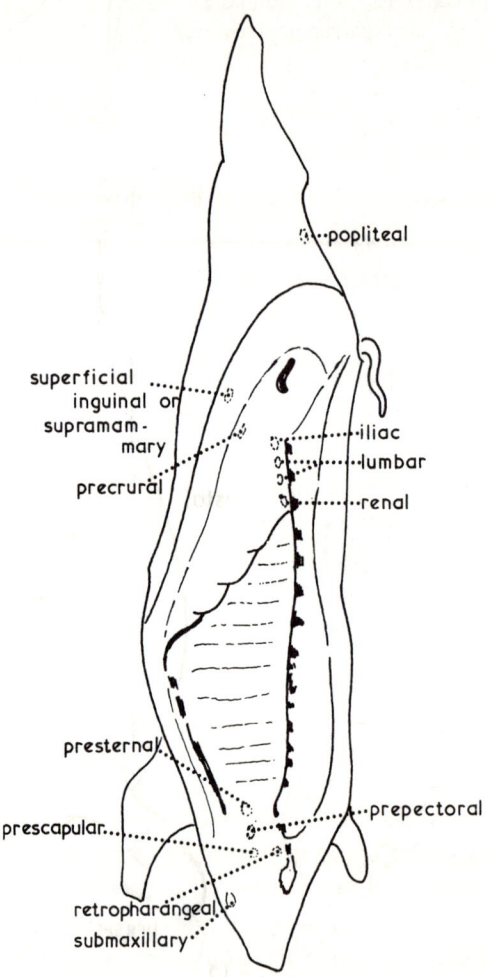

popliteal

superficial
inguinal or
supramam-
mary

precrural

iliac

lumbar

renal

presternal

prescapular

prepectoral

retropharangeal
submaxillary

Figure 13

The spleen.

Another organ intimately connected with the circulatory system must receive separate mention. This is the spleen. It is to be found on the left side of the abdominal cavity, and in cattle it lies to the front

of the rumen.   Its purpose is not fully understood, and life is possible
without a spleen, but it would appear to have the following functions:
(1) it plays a part in the formation of white blood cells, (2) it destroys some old red blood cells and to some extent may supply new
ones, and (3) it acts as a spongy store for red blood cells while the
animal is at rest.   When more oxygen is needed it contracts, releasing
cells and their haemoglobin potential into the circulation.

The formation of blood cells

Most of the cells in the blood are formed in the bone marrow, the
remainder, the lymphocytes are formed in the lymph glands.   The
common origin of the cells in the *myeloid* tissue of the marrow is a
cell known as a *haemocytoblast*.   In simple terms this means a blood
cell embryo.   The red blood cells are formed in vast numbers in bone
marrow, starting like all cells with a nucleus, and gradually losing
this in the process of formation.   At any one time there are numerous
red blood cells waiting to be taken up in the blood.   In case of need
they can be released in large numbers.

Many types of white cells are also produced in the marrow; these,
as explained, are capable of defending the body by ingesting bacteria
and other invaders of the blood.   They too increase greatly in numbers during the course of bacterial infection.

Examination of the blood

Blood may be readily obtained and examined under the microscope
or in the laboratory, therefore the making and investigation of
disease using blood smears is an important part of field diagnosis.

Firstly, the number of red blood cells in the sample is important.
This may be tested by comparing the packed cell volume, that is the
precipitation of the cells after the sample has been centrifuged, with
the normal value for the species.   Then the shape of the red blood
cells, and whether they are young or old.   Also whether parasites are
to be found either in the plasma or in the cells.   The number of
white cells may also be a good indication of the presence of infection,
since, as explained, they enter the blood in great numbers when the
body is threatened.

Since the spleen acts as a reservoir of red blood cells one of the easiest ways to detect protozoal parasites in blood cells is to take a spleen smear.   Unfortunately this technique can only be applied in the dead animal, but it is a method of examination which should always be carried out if blood parasites are suspected.

THE DIGESTIVE SYSTEM

The process of digestion is the process by which food substances are broken down into a form in which they may be absorbed into the animal body.   In essence the process may be thought of simply as a means of bringing quite complex, often insoluble compounds, into a form in which they may be made soluble or their component molecules broken down so that they may pass tissue barriers.   The digestive system is therefore the series of tubes and containers which hold the food on its way from mouth to anus while energy-giving and building materials are drawn from it and absorbed.   In short, solid materials are taken in at the mouth, broken down in the digestive tract, divested of substance useful to the body, and excreted at the other end.

All animal food is a combination of water (H_2O) and carbon dioxide (C_2O) with variable quantities of nitrogen and minerals.   The chain starts with the manufacture of organic substances by plants from water and carbon dioxide using the energy of the sun through chlorophyll.   Some animals have adapted their digestive system to the storage and breakdown of vegetable matter, and the absorption from their intestines of solutions containing the products of this process.   These are the herbivores, and their specialized diets are obtained by grazing or browsing on products of plants—that is roots, tubers, leaves, flowers, fruits and sometimes bark and smaller twigs.

Plant foods are very bulky because they contain a large amount of indigestible fibre, so the herbivore has to provide a means of storage somewhere in the digestive tract to hold quantities of vegetable matter before digestion.   Ruminants are the most highly developed herbivores, and possess a large sack-like container, divided into three unequally sized compartments, lying between the end of the *oesophagus* or gullet and the true stomach or *abomasum*.   The largest compartment is known as the *rumen*, and the two others as the *reticulum* and the *omasum*. Cattle are typical examples of animals with ruminant digestion, although sheep and goats have similar systems. Herbivores like the horse and the rabbit have developed a large *caecum* or capacious large intestine in order to hold bulky plant food. The caecum is a blind sack found between the small and large intestines and known as the appendix in man. In both these animals it is greatly enlarged, but the impression is gained that this system of plant material digestion is not as efficient as that in ruminants since the droppings, particularly of horses, often contain considerable quantities of undigested vegetable matter. Bacteria are needed in the rumen, caecum or large intestine in order to break down cellulose.

During the process of evolution other animals have found an easier way of getting their food than spending hours each day eating grass. They get what they need by killing and eating the herbivores. These predators need a far shorter intestine than their prey since the food they eat is already in a suitable form for mammalian digestion. They do, however, tend to have stomachs which are capable of great dilation so that they can hold in them large quantities of meat, so reducing the number of meals they would need if the food was all to be taken in small amounts.

The digestive system of the ox

The adaptation to a vegetable diet starts with the mouth. Cattle graze by cutting grass off with their front teeth or incisors, against the hard palate in the upper jaw, and using their tongues to draw the stalks together. A great quantity of watery *saliva* is secreted by the *salivary glands* in the mouth of ruminants. This creates a digestive action through an enzyme called *ptyalin* but is also useful in lubricating the food on its way to the rumen where it is stored. After grazing for some time, the animal rests and regurgitates the food from the rumen back into the mouth in convenient boluses. These are ground between the back teeth, or molars, which have been adapted into grinding plates. The jaws have also become adapted to permit considerable lateral movement so enabling the lower jaw molars to slide across those of the upper jaw.

Behind the bulb of the tongue at the back of the mouth is the *pharynx*; this is a muscular chamber from which both the *trachea*, or breathing tube, and the oesophagus arise. Guarding the trachea, and

preventing food from getting into the lungs, is the *epiglottis*.   This is
a leaf-like structure which can be easily seen in the dead animal, and
sometimes felt in the live when searching for an obstruction at the

STORAGE OF FOOD
—THE STOMACH

Simple Stomach—the dog

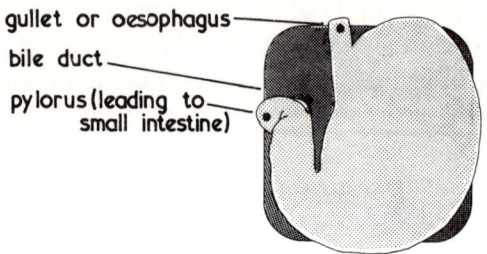

Complex Stomach the ox

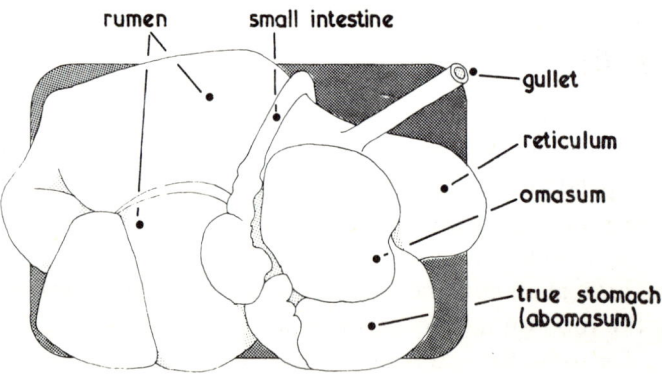

Figure 14

back of the mouth in a choking cow.   Potatoes or other roots may
get stuck at the pharynx or at the start of the oesophagus, and in
some cases may not only choke but asphyxiate the animal by restricting breathing.

The function of the rumen, reticulum and omasum have been
explained but their linings are very distinctive.   At the point where

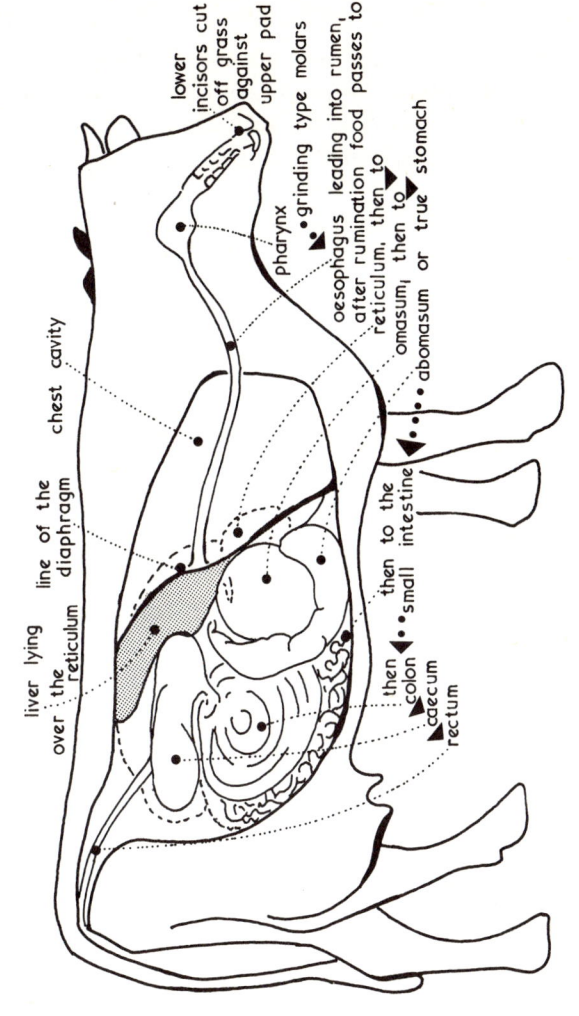

THE DIGESTIVE TRACT OF THE COW

lower incisors cut off grass against upper pad

pharynx

grinding type molars

oesophagus leading into rumen, after rumination food passes to reticulum, then to

omasum, then to

abomasum or true stomach

liver lying over the reticulum

line of the diaphragm

chest cavity

then to the small intestine

then colon

caecum

rectum

Figure 15

the oesophagus enters the rumen there is a muscular tube known as the oesophageal groove. It can be opened or closed as circumstances dictate. When closed it allows water and fine ruminated food to pass directly into the omasum and from there into the abomasum or true stomach. When it is open, food passes into the rumen. In the suckling calf the oesophageal groove is closed and until weaning the young animal is not a true ruminant. The contents of the rumen are normally quite fluid, but those of the reticulum and omasum are much drier. It is probable that water is mainly absorbed from these two containers.

The abomasum leads into the small intestine, and the small intestine into the large intestine. Gastric juices from the abomasum start a process of digestion which is continued in the small intestine. Because the process of break-down of fine food particles into small soluble compounds takes some time and requires close mixing of the enzymes with the food, the small intestine is very long and very narrow. In the ox it is some 45 m (130 ft) long. Digestion in the small intestine is assisted by secretion from the *pancreas* (a large ducted gland lying in a loop of small intestine) and also by the extracts released into it through the *bile duct.* The products of the bile duct arise from the liver, and have a distinctive colour seen in the colour of droppings. The large intestine or *colon* arises at the point where the caecum also arises. The caecum is some 60 cm (2 ft) long in cattle and the colon about 10 m (35 ft). Water is extracted from the waste substances in the colon and the relatively dry dung is extruded from the anus. Cattle appear to have less control over the release of *faecal* matter or dung than some other animals.

The function of the liver and pancreas

The liver is the largest gland in the body and is in fact the centre of the animal's metabolism. The food substances collected from the intestinal tract by diffusion into the blood vessels are taken to the liver where they are changed into proteins, fats and carbohydrates of direct value to the individual concerned. The liver has therefore many functions but the three most important are:
   (1) The storage of animal starch or glycogen.
   (2) The breakdown of red blood cells when they can no longer

perform their function. This results in the excretion of bile into the intestine where it assists pancreatic enzymes in digestion.

(3) The filtering of waste products out of the blood and their conversion to urea, which is transmitted to the kidneys in the blood stream, and eliminated in the urine.

It is apparent therefore that damage to the liver affects the whole body, and that where a disease which results in an increased destruction of red blood cells also has a profound effect on the ability of the liver to function normally. The parasites known as liver flukes

THE DIGESTIVE SYSTEM OF THE PIG (AN OMNIVORE)

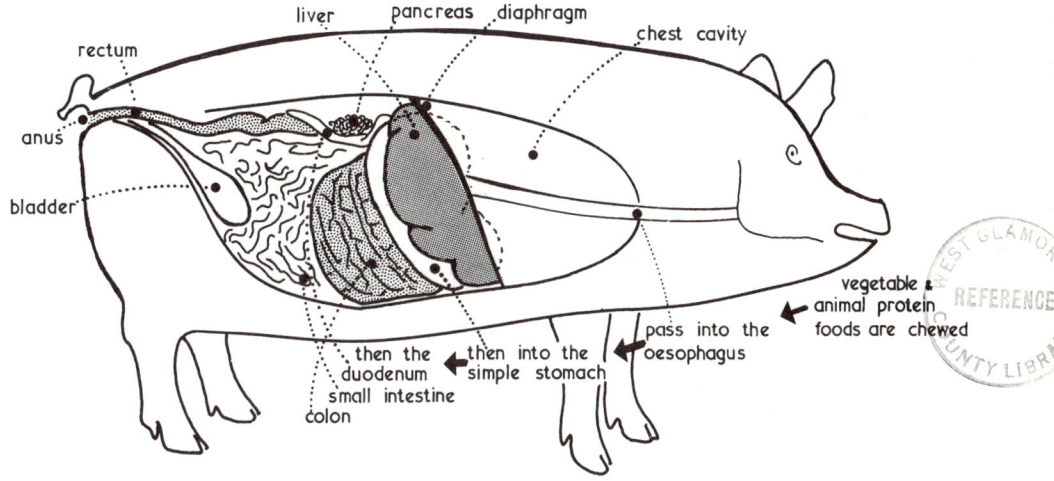

Figure 16

(*Fasciola* species) do particular damage by migrating through liver tissue and destroying it. Any profound change in metabolism caused by disease is often reflected in the appearance of the liver, and a liver so damaged may take some time to recover. However, the liver is very large and sufficient tissue will remain to support function, even in cases where it would seem that much of it has been damaged beyond repair.

In essence the liver is a filter of the blood, the manufacturer of substances used in body processes and the eliminator of waste products.

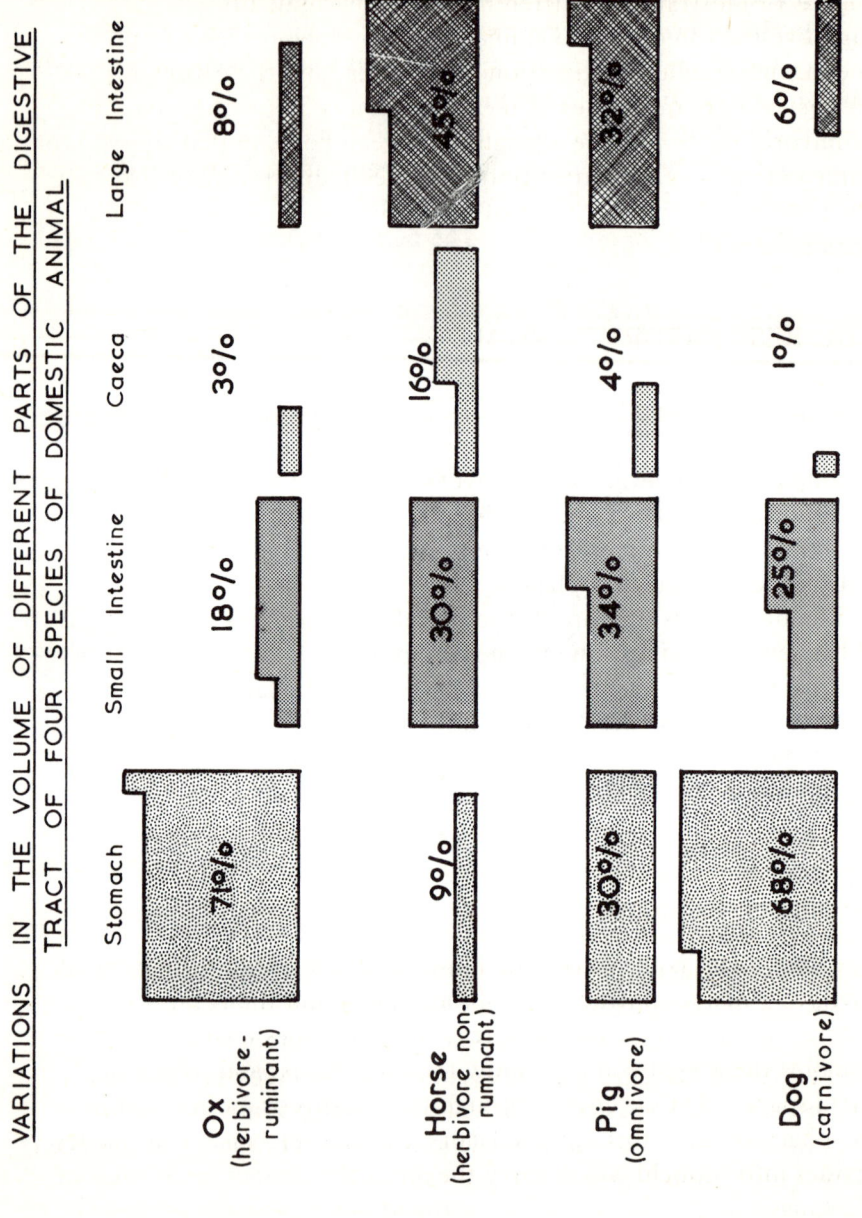

VARIATIONS IN THE VOLUME OF DIFFERENT PARTS OF THE DIGESTIVE TRACT OF FOUR SPECIES OF DOMESTIC ANIMAL

Stomach   Small Intestine   Caeca   Large Intestine

Ox (herbivore-ruminant)   71%   18%   3%   8%

Horse (herbivore non-ruminant)   9%   30%   16%   45%

Pig (omnivore)   30%   34%   4%   32%

Dog (carnivore)   68%   25%   1%   6%

Figure 17

The digestive tracts of omnivores and carnivores

Figure 17 illustrates the differences in the weights of each part of the digestive tract in domestic animals. The herbivores have to provide the means of cellulose digestion by bacteria, and the carnivores storage of large quantities of meat between infrequent meals. The omnivores try to provide a balance between both, in that they do to some extent have the capacity to digest cellulose but they also have the need to take in quantities of meat to make up their metabolic requirements.

THE RESPIRATORY SYSTEM

The epiglottis is the leaf-like piece of cartilage which stands upright between the back of the tongue and the entrance to the *larynx*. During the act of swallowing, it works as a valve which seals off the entrance to the larynx and wind-pipe. Food and liquids on being swallowed pass directly from the back of the tongue over the epiglottis and into the oesophagus.

The pharynx is the throat, the chamber at the back of the mouth. It has seven openings: one from the mouth; one to the gullet or oesophagus; two from the nasal chambers; one to the larynx and two from the ears. The Eustachian tubes open onto the *pharynx*.

The larynx is the voice box, placed at the top of the trachea. It acts as a valve by regulating the air intake and also by trapping any foreign particles that may be inhaled.

Respiration and inspiration

The diaphragm is the muscle dividing the chest from the abdominal cavity. When it contracts the ribs are raised and the volume of the pleural cavity in the chest is increased. Air rushes into the lungs to equalize the pressure and to allow the lungs to expand to fill the extra space. The air enters through the nostrils or mouth first into the pharynx, then through the larynx into the trachea. The trachea divides into bronchi which carry the air in the air sacs or alveolae of the lungs.

The pharynx and larynx both have very sensitive nerve endings. If these nerve endings are irritated by the entry of dust or other particles, a coughing reflex occurs.   The larynx supports the vocal cords and leads into the trachea.   The *trachea* or windpipe is a flexible tube which is prevented from collapsing by incomplete rings of cartilage. The rings are joined by muscle and the tube is lined by a mucous membrane kept moist by mucus secreting cells.

The trachea runs from the larynx down the centre of the lower part of the neck, enters the thorax or chest cavity and ends by dividing into 2 or 3 bronchi (2 in the dog and horse; 3 in the ox, sheep and pig).   The bronchi in their upper part are of similar cartilaginous structure to the trachea.   But they soon split up into *bronchioles* which lose much of their cartilage as they divide and subdivide, becoming smaller and smaller until they end up in the air sacs of the lungs which are arranged around the ends of the smallest bronchioles.

The air sacs have very thin walls around which many capillaries (tiny blood vessels) form a close meshwork.   These capillaries are separated from the air in the sacs by a very thin layer of protoplasm through which a gaseous exchange is effected.   Carbonic acid gas is passed from the blood in the capillaries to the air sacs and then breathed out.   At the same time, the inhaled oxygen is taken up by the red blood cells from the fresh air in the air sacs.

The result of the repeated branching of the air tubes in the lung is to bring the largest possible surface of blood under the air in the air sacs.   In man, about 230 m^2 (1500 ft^2) of blood surface are exposed to the air in this way at each inspiration.   In other words, the blood coming from the pulmonary artery is spread out onto the equivalent of a film of blood, one cell thick, covering the floor space of a room 23 m (75 ft) long and 6 m (20 ft) wide; it is then gathered up again in the pulmonary vein and returned to the heart.

Expiration

Expiration is caused by the diaphragm relaxing, allowing the ribs to fall thus compressing the lungs and forcing the air from them.

Respiratory rate

Respiration is carried out by voluntary muscles controlled by reflexes over which the animal can exert a certain amount of control.   The number of respirations per minute varies in different animals. Generally, the smaller the animal, the greater the rate.

Man:	14–18 per minute	Pig:	10–15 per minute
Horse:	8–10 per minute	Dog:	15–20 per minute
Ox:	12–15 per minute	Fowl:	About 60 per minute
Sheep:	12–20 per minute		

The pleural membranes

The pleural membranes cover the inner surface of the pleural cavity and surround the lungs. Normally there is a small amount of serous fluid between them which increases with pleurisy (inflammation).

Voice production

Voice production in mammals is carried out by the larynx, which has two vocal cords in a 'V' shape and these cords, together with the pharynx, the mouth and nasal chambers, all assist in producing the different noises made by animals.

THE EXCRETORY SYSTEM

Two sorts of substances are voided from the body. No animal has the ability to select only that food which will suffice for its immediate needs, therefore it adopts a more sensible procedure. It takes in as much food as it can while it is available, and more of that food which appeals to it. The result is that the indigestible part, together with food which passes through the intestine too quickly to be properly absorbed, is voided at the anus. This is the dung or faeces, and it is coloured by breakdown products of metabolism produced by the liver, and dribbled into the intestine through the bile duct.

The other waste products pass through the kidneys, after process in the body. It must not be forgotten however that carbon dioxide is also voided through the lungs, and that water and sodium chloride are excreted in sweat through the skin.

THE KIDNEY

Kidney of the Ox

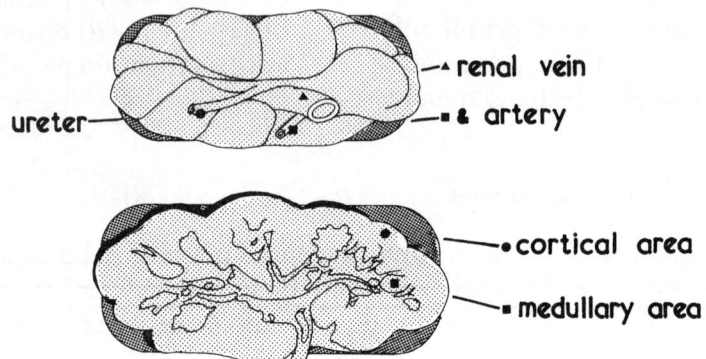

ureter — — renal vein
— & artery

— cortical area
— medullary area

Kidney of the Pig

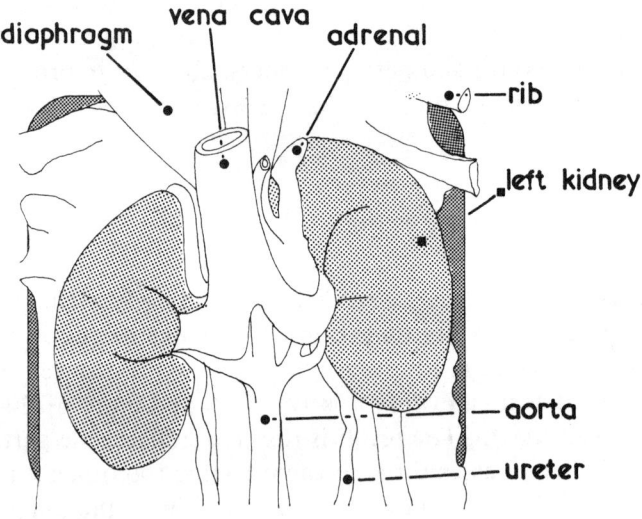

diaphragm   vena cava   adrenal
— rib
— left kidney
— aorta
— ureter

Figure 18

The kidneys

The kidneys in mammals are found lying on each side of the spinal cord in the lumbar region, and sometimes loosely attached to the body wall but near enough to the bone structure of the vertebrae to receive protection against blows.   The form and shape of the kidneys vary from species to species but their function remains the same.

In cut section, a kidney is seen to consist of a dark coloured outer zone called the *cortex*, surrounding a lighter zone known as the *medulla*.   The cortex contains great numbers of *glomeruli* or little capsules served by blood vessels, those leading into the glomerulus being smaller than those leaving it.   This is because the main function of the capsule is to take water from the blood and start it on its journey down from the capsule through the medulla into the ureter.

THE   GLOMERULUS   OR   EXCRETORY MECHANISM   OF   THE   KIDNEY

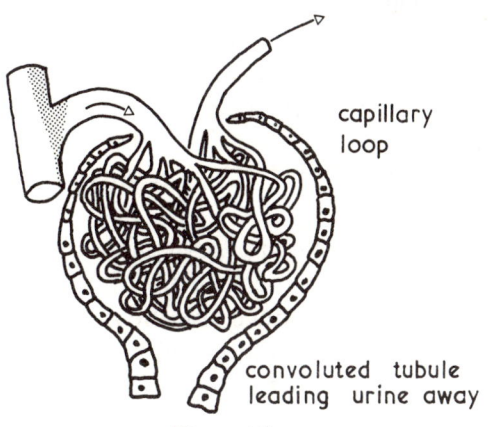

capillary loop

convoluted   tubule leading   urine   away

Figure 19

Each capsule ends therefore in a tiny tube, which, like a stream lead- ing into a river, joins those of its neighbours to form larger and larger vessels until finally the main tube or ureter is reached.   The ureter joins the bladder where urine is stored, and, as already mentioned, the bladder is closed by a sphincter muscle which is under both voluntary and involuntary control.   In the female the bladder opens into the vagina, and in the male, into the penis.

The secretion of water by the glomeruli of the kidney, or by evaporation through the skin provides a means of controlling body temperature.   In hot weather water is secreted as sweat to reduce body temperature, and in cold weather through the kidney to con- serve it.   Nitrogenous wastes in the form of urea, and excess electro- lytes pass into the bladder in solution.

The functions of the kidney

No organ in the body has one restricted function; usually it contains the means of initiating and controlling a variety of useful properties, and the kidneys are no exception. The functions of the kidney may be catalogued as follows, but again beware of regarding each of these functions as operating in isolation from the others. Most of the properties are inter-related.

(1) The kidneys conserve water, they prevent it being lost in too great a quantity, yet ensure that the concentration of the blood is maintained.

(2) In removing water they retain larger molecules like glucose and amino acids, although both in excess may be excreted.

(3) They remove nitrogenous waste which arises as a result of protein metabolism. This is mainly done in the form of urea, which can rise to dangerous and toxic heights when the glomeruli of the kidneys are damaged.

(4) They maintain the pH of the body fluids by eliminating excess hydrogen ions.

(5) They eliminate some complex organic substances which arise either by absorption or by manufacture within the body.

(6) Two hormones are produced by the kidney. One of these is important in the regulation of blood cell formation, and the other is renin which affects the production of *aldosterone*. Aldosterone is produced by the cortex of the adrenal glands and is concerned with the maintainance of the pH of the blood. Its absence is followed by loss of blood sodium, chloride and bicarbonate, and by a rise in the level of potassium. The adrenals are found in close proximity to the kidneys, one on either side of the body.

Despite this long catalogue of functions the point to remember is that the kidneys control the level of water in the body. In extreme desiccation they can never cut off urine secretion entirely because of the necessity to remove urea and other harmful substances from the blood, but they do their best. In the absence of sufficient water the urine is concentrated and becomes a deeper yellow in colour.

It follows from all this that the health of the body can be determined to some extent from examining urine. When parasites which destroy red cells are present in the blood the urine turns red with haemoglobin or yellow with jaundice. When glucose is present in excess, as in a disease known as *diabetes*, it too can be measured in urine.   When kidneys are damaged by injury or disease amino acid retention is affected and protein substances may pass out.   Like other body fluids urine samples may provide a means of determining the state of health.

THE NERVOUS SYSTEM

The nervous system operates from the brain and spinal cord.   It receives messages from the sense organs, the skin and tissues, and transmits calls for action to the muscles.   The nerve cells are all contained in the brain and the messages move along filaments known as *axons* which stretch out and form junctions in all parts of the body.

The efficiency of the nerves depends on two characteristics of living tissue.   One is the ability to appreciate irritation, and the other is to transmit that irritation as a stimulus.

As forms of life expanded and multicellular animals became more complicated, rudimentary nerve cells emerged to enable the increasingly complex body movements to be coordinated.   Gradually sense organs developed to receive information from the world outside the organism, and the central nervous system formed to interpret this information and to produce a reaction to it.   The first requirement was to survive, and so pain stimuli developed and avoidance movements took place.   The second and concurrent requirement was the seeking of food so automatic responses developed to make food easier to find and capture.   Finally the ultimate occurred, the brain became organized to the point where actions could be planned into the future, and then man was born.

The receptor organs

There are five senses.   All are important to maintain an animal in its environment, but different species place different emphasis on the senses that they have developed for their own particular circumstances.   Sight is important to all domestic animals, but it is clear that they do not all see objects in the same way that man does. Predatory animals like cats and dogs see forward with both eyes, but dogs retain more lateral vision than do cats.   Both cattle and horses

THE NEURON OR NERVE CELL

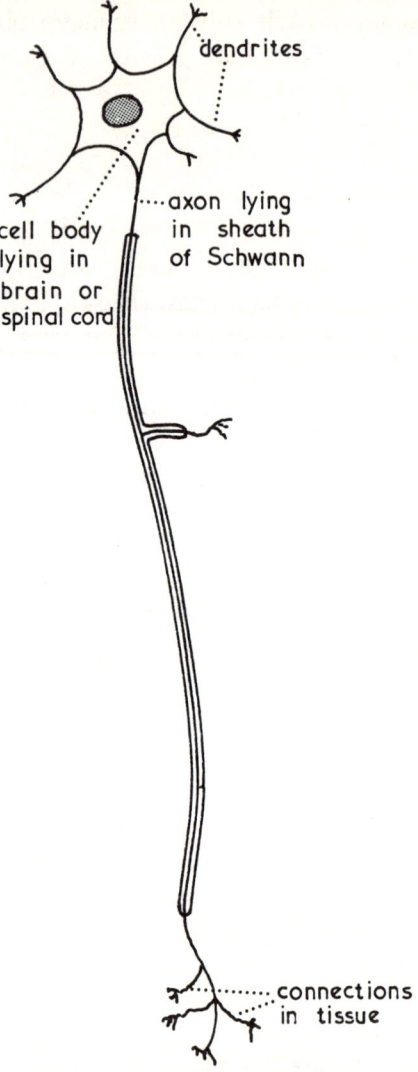

Figure 20

value lateral vision, but horses see further to the side and behind than do cattle.

Hearing is acute in both dogs and cats, not quite so acute in cattle and horses. Animals however retain a different range of sounds than is the case in man. Taste also differs for obvious reasons; herbivores prefer vegetable tastes and carnivores meat tastes. Touch is much the same in all animals; but man probably has a greater appreciation of differences in surface texture than many animals, because he has fingers, whereas animals have feet covered by horn, thick skin or fur.

It is however, in the sense of smell that animals differ most from man. By simple observation it is clear that animals appreciate a whole world opened to them by their acute ability to distinguish smells, which is entirely denied to man. Some might say that man has exchanged a sense of smell for an ability to calculate.

Reflex actions

Certain actions monitored well down the spinal chord solicit immediate unthought response. These are the reflex actions. Recoil from pain is one such.

The structure of the brain

No attempt is made here to detail the various parts of the brain but the main divisions may be seen in the diagram. It is important however, to have some idea of the various functions of the sections of the brain because many are referred to in the literature.

The cerebrum

The cerebrum is divided into two equal parts or hemispheres, and is the part of the brain concerned with the recognition of the environment and the determination of the actions necessary to take advantage of it. This description has a simple sound but the reality is by no means simple, and involves the whole concept of conscious thought. We cannot know how far an animal can think but it is clear that it can develop learning processes. What it does not have is prolonged and complex memory, although memory is clearly retained better in some individuals than others.

The *olfactory lobes* are found one on each side and in front of the hemispheres of the cerebrum. They are concerned with the sense of smell.

The cerebellum

This lies behind the cerebrum and near to the posterior part of the brain, it is largely concerned with the coordination of movement.

The optic nerves

The importance of sight to land animals is demonstrated by the size of the optic nerves and their close proximity to the brain. Messages from the eyes must be reflected almost instantaneously in the brain, and action may be organized all the more quickly because of this.

The pituitary gland

This is the most important ductless gland in the body. It is divided into two parts, a forepart or the anterior pituitary, and the rearpart or posterior pituitary. Reproductive hormones regulating the female sexual cycle originate in the anterior pituitary, while the posterior pituitary has function in connection with the stimulation of growth. The diagram summarizes these.

The internal anatomy of the brain

The so-called grey matter is on the outside of the brain and is composed of the nerve cells whose prominences, immensely enlarged and elongated, extrude from the white matter in the centre. Each one may be likened to a very thin telephone wire connecting a cell which is in the grey matter. Each cell forms many connections with its neighbours and an elaborate and complex computer is formed which can monitor and respond to impulses received from the outer world.

The meninges

These are the thin membranes covering the brain and spinal cord. Between the lining of the cranium and the covering of the brain is a small amount of fluid in which the brain floats.

Cranial nerves

There are 12 main cranial nerves (nerves of the head) which start in pairs from the brain and go to the right and left side of the body. They branch off to the various organs and are given different names according to their function.

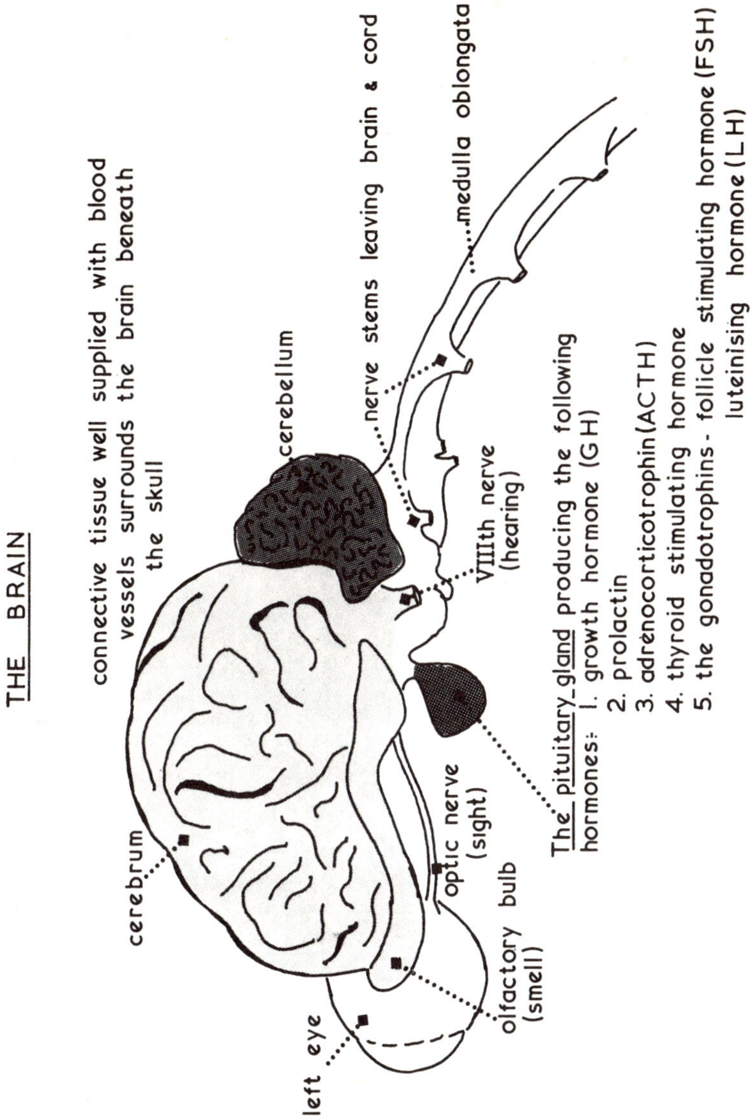

THE BRAIN

connective tissue well supplied with blood
vessels surrounds the brain beneath
the skull

medulla oblongata

nerve stems leaving brain & cord

cerebellum

VIIIth nerve
(hearing)

The pituitary gland producing the following
hormones: 1. growth hormone (GH)
2. prolactin
3. adrenocorticotrophin (ACTH)
4. thyroid stimulating hormone
5. the gonadotrophins - follicle stimulating hormone (FSH)
luteinising hormone (LH)

cerebrum

optic nerve
(sight)

olfactory bulb
(smell)

left eye

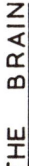

Figure 21

The hippocampus

When the brain is sectioned the hippocampus will be found lying under the ventricles.

THE EYE IN SECTION

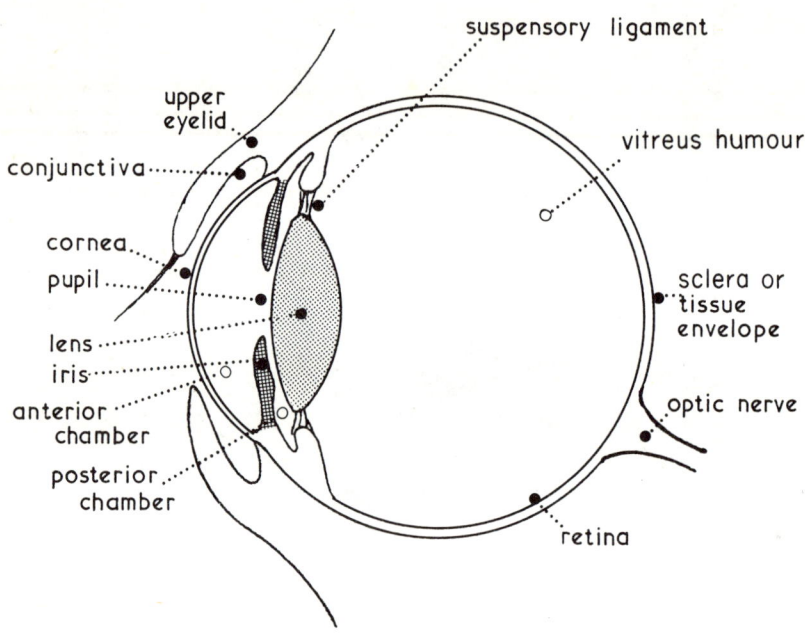

Movement of the eyeball is by muscles attached to the sclera

Figure 22

Medulla oblongata

This is the part of the nervous system lying between the forebrain and the spinal cord.   It controls respiration, the heart beat, and the digestive secretions and movements.   The spinal cord is a continuation of the medulla.   Unlike the brain, the white matter of the spinal cord is on the outside, the grey matter on the inside.   The white matter contains nerve fibres linking together the various parts of the central nervous system. It gives off about 42 paired nerves, one for each side of the body.

From these branch nerves such as the radial, median and ulna to the fore limb and the femoral and sciatic to the hind limb.

It is interesting to note that the right side of the brain controls the left side of the body, the left side controls the right side of the body.

The eye

The eye is specially adapted to receive visual images and to pass them through the optic nerve to the brain. It is constructed like a camera. In the centre of the globular eyeball is a lens. The eyeball is made of a tough, white, fibrous coat called the sclera. The front part of the eyeball, the cornea, is transparent and allows the light to pass the lens and through there to the retina, the screen at the back of the eyeball where the optic nerve originates.

From the bony socket in the skull, six muscles are attached to the eyeball to make it movable.

The conjunctiva, a delicate membrane lining the eyelids and continued over the front of the cornea, is normally pale pink but in disease conditions it often changes colour.

The eyelashes, the eyelids and the lachrymal glands, which produce a watery secretion that bathes the front of the eye, all act as protection against dust and foreign bodies that might otherwise damage the cornea.

The lachrymal fluid drains into a tiny duct in the inner corner of the eye and from there into the nasal chambers. This helps to carry away dust or grit that may lodge on the surface of the conjunctiva.

THE REPRODUCTIVE SYSTEM

All young animals originate in one cell; in the higher animals this is formed by the union of a male sperm cell with the female cell or ovum. Both the male and female cells carry half a nucleus to their union, and by the fusion of these two halves a new organism is created which combines genetic characteristics from both its mother and father, or in animal terms, its dam and sire.

The process of reproduction in mammals has evolved to make sure that the young animal shall develop during its most vulnerable and helpless period in the body of its mother. When it is large enough it is pushed into the world, and develops further under the protection of one or more parents until it may fend for itself.

The organs of reproduction ensure that sperm and the ovum shall meet with a good chance of fertilization, while giving the *embryo* protection. A very complex mechanism is required to make sure that this timing is carried out correctly and with the minimum of waste.

The male sex organs

The testicles are the male sex glands which produce the sperm and some of the seminal fluid in which the sex cells are conveyed into the female organs. They rest outside the body in a sac of skin known as the *scrotum*, which has two compartments, one for each gland. Each testicle is surrounded by a tough connective tissue membrane known as the *tunica vaginalis* which is continuous with that of the *peritoneum*, through the *inguinal groove*. In the tube thus formed lies the spermatic cord. This consists of the narrow tube used to convey sperm and some seminal fluid and known as the *ductus deferens*, and the blood vessels and nerves which supply the testicles. Sperm is stored in the seminal vesicles which lie near the exit of the bladder in the bull, and further fluid is supplied by the *prostate gland*, also found in the same area. The sperm duct passes through the centre of the *penis* in which it is surrounded by spongy tissue capable of erection through suffusion with quantities of blood.

The stimulus for erection and for mounting and penetration of the female arises from the female, within whose body a complex series of hormonal interactions initiates the sexual cycle.

The female sex organs

Each mammalian female has two ovaries lying one on each side of the body, protected by the pelvic girdle. The ovaries are suspended within the abdominal cavity by a ligament known as the *ovarian ligament*. Near to each ovary is the entrance to the uterus or womb. The wide cup-like structure near the ovary leads into a narrow tube on each side, called the *fallopian tube*, which leads into a horn of the

REPRODUCTIVE ORGANS OF CATTLE

The Male

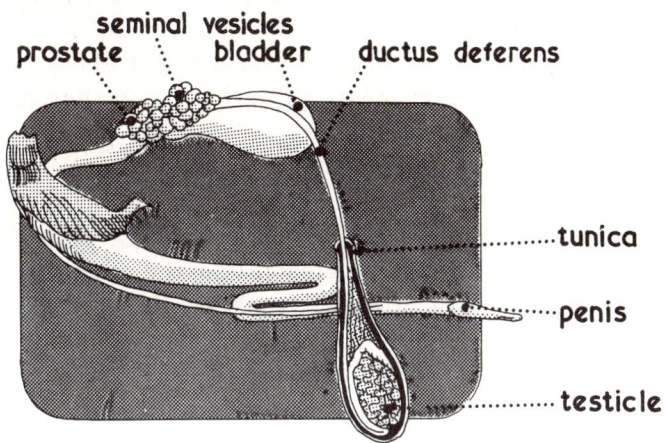

seminal vesicles
prostate   bladder   ductus deferens

tunica

penis

testicle

The Female

cotyledons

fallopian tubes

ovary

uterus

cervix

vagina(cut open)

opening of ureter

vulva

Figure 23

uterus.   The horns of the uterus open into the body of that organ which is separated from the *vagina* by a sphincter muscle known as the *cervix*, and opens to the exterior at the *vulva*.

In addition to the primary sexual organs the female also possesses a number of milk or *mammary* glands which feed the young animal after birth. The number of mammary glands varies with each species of animal and is to a certain extent regulated by the number of young normally born at the one time. The anatomy of the mammary gland of the cow is shown in the diagram but there are certain differences in other species of animal.

Carnivores like dogs and cats give birth to young at a very much earlier stage in the life of the fetus than is the case in herbivores. They produce more young, and it is of interest that the number of streak canals at the base of the teat is greater than the single canal found almost universally among ruminants. Pigs also produce a number of young and have the same number of mammary glands as bitches.

The sexual cycle

The sexual cycle is a pattern of behaviour, initiated by the female, and guided by hormones. It results in the sperm fertilizing the ovum within the female reproductive tract at a time when conditions are such that the resulting embryo can be nourished to grow into a young animal.

The hormones which guide the cycle in the female arise as a result of the stimulation of the pituitary gland by message from the hypothalamus. The pituitary hormones interact with other hormones originating in the ovary, or, later in pregnancy, with those arising from the uterus or from the placenta within which the fetus lies.

The cycle is designed therefore to result in pregnancy; but should pregnancy not occur, then a variable pattern takes place depending on the species which is studied.

The signs of heat

To some extent these vary between species, but by and large consist of: swelling of the vulva, discharge from the vagina, restlessness, mounting of other animals and standing to be mounted. Heat periods of the domestic species are shown in the appendix.

The gestation period

This is the length of time for which the mother carries the young. It varies in the different species.

Cow: 280 days (average)   about 9 months
Mare: 340 days (average)   about 11 months
Ewe: 150 days (average)   about 5 months
Sow: 115 days (average)   about 4 months
Bitch: 62 days (average)   about 2 months

The hormonal control of the cycle

Only the natural state is considered here, and only in very general terms.   Each species differs in detail as explained in the section on behaviour but all animals have the same basic hormonal pattern.

In *anoestrus* the ovary is inactive and the genital tract is in a resting phase.   The female shows no interest in the male, and no interest in young animals.   In other words the sexual and maternal influences are at their lowest point.

The weather at the breeding time of the year probably causes stimuli from the hypothalamus to increase the activity of the pituitary gland.   This gland constantly secretes two hormones in differing concentrations depending on the stimuli it receives.   These hormones are *FSH* or follicle stimulating hormone and *LH* or luteinizing hormone.

Activated by the hypothalamus the pituitary increases the amount of FSH it is secreting.   This has an effect on the ovary by causing the follicles which contain the ova or eggs to enlarge.   As they get bigger they move towards the surface of the ovary and they start to secrete another hormone, *oestrogen* or female sexual hormone, which has the effect of preparing the sexual tissues of the female for the process of *copulation*, and for the ready transport of the sperms up the uterine tract into the fallopian tubes where they will encounter and fertilize the ova.

Oestrogen therefore produces enlargement of the vulva and increased secretion in the vagina, as well as relaxation of its walls and relaxation of the cervix.   It also causes the female to be more interested in the male.   This preparation to the act of mating is known as *pro-oestrus*.   As the follicle reaches the surface of the ovary and ripens to the point of being ready to burst and release the egg, the level of oestrogen rises to the extent that it has an effect on the pituitary.   This effect is a reduction of excretion of FSH, and an increase in the production of LH.

LH is responsible for the bursting of the follicle, the release of the

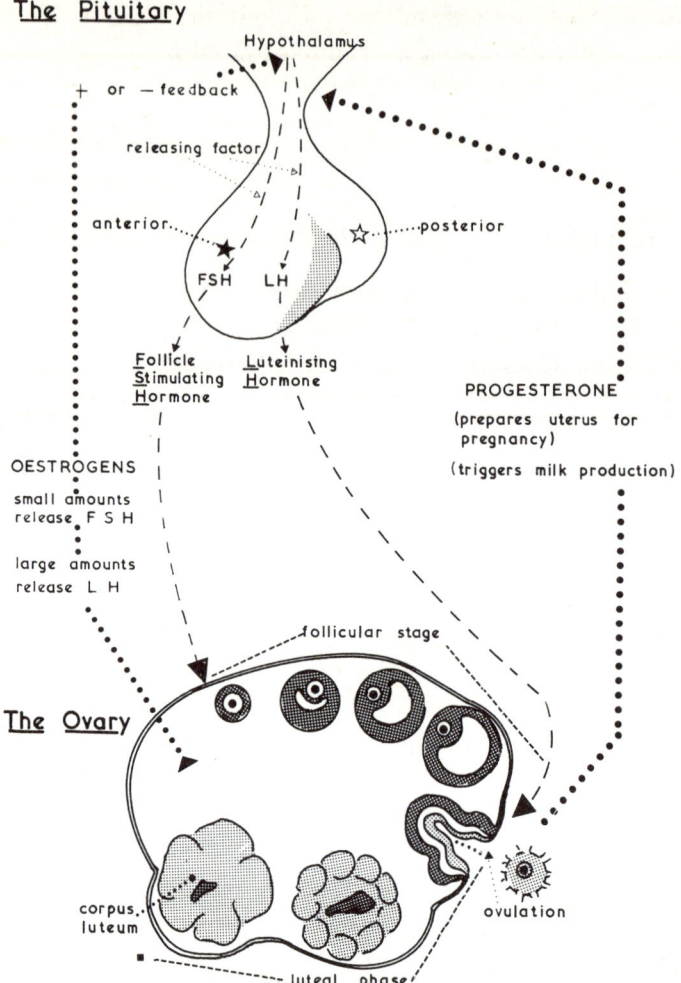

HORMONAL CONTROL OF OVULATION IN MAMMALS

Figure 24

ovum, and the formation of the burst follicle into a large yellow body which is called the *corpus luteum*. The time of greatest sexual activity, which corresponds with the highest level of oestrogen, results in the acceptance of the male by the female. This is the period known as *oestrus*. It may or may not coincide with ovulation, or the release of the ova, in some animals it does and in some it does not. In the cow ovulation occurs some 48 hours after oestrus, in the cat and rabbit the stimulus for ovulation is provided by *coitus*.

Hormonal control of pregnancy

A choice of two alternatives now occurs.   The corpus luteum secretes
a substance known as *progesterone*; this hormone has the effect of
preparing the uterus to receive the fertilized ovum.   If the ovum
becomes fertilized, moves down the fallopian tube and becomes
secured to the wall of the uterus, pregnancy has occurred.   The
process of attachment to the wall of the uterus is known as *nidation*.
Pregnancy continues partly as a result of the action of the progesterone secreted by the corpus luteum, and partly as a result of progesterone secreted by the placenta of the growing *embryo*.   The
placenta is the means by which the young animal obtains nutriment
from its mother while it is in the uterus.   The embryo grows into a
fetus and develops to the point of time when it is ready to enter the
outside world by the process of birth or *parturition*.   During the
development, progesterone, and another hormone known as *prolactin*,
begin to act on the mammary glands or udder to prepare for the production of milk to nourish the newly born animal.   It is thought that
the action of birth is started by hormones (probably from the adrenal
gland) of the fetus acting on the hormonal mechanisms of its
mother.

At the time of birth, the mammary glands contain a substance
hardly recognizable as milk but with special properties.   It is known
as *colostrum* or first milk and is yellow in colour.   It contains special
protein substances known as *immunoglobulins*, which help the young
animal to overcome infection in the first days of life.

The cycle in the absence of pregnancy

In the event of fertilization not taking place the corpus luteum gradually declines in size and the sexual organs return to their resting stage.
The details of the way this process is accomplished varies between
species.   Cattle have a three week interval between cycles so that the
period of sexual inactivity in the absence of pregnancy is short.
Horses have the same type of polycycle but exhibit a seasonal pattern.
Thus the cycles start in spring and cease in late summer.   Sows cycle
repeatedly when they are not weaning young.   Cats are seasonally
polycyclic like the horse, and bitches have one cycle at very infrequent
intervals.

THE   MAMMARY   GLAND OF THE COW

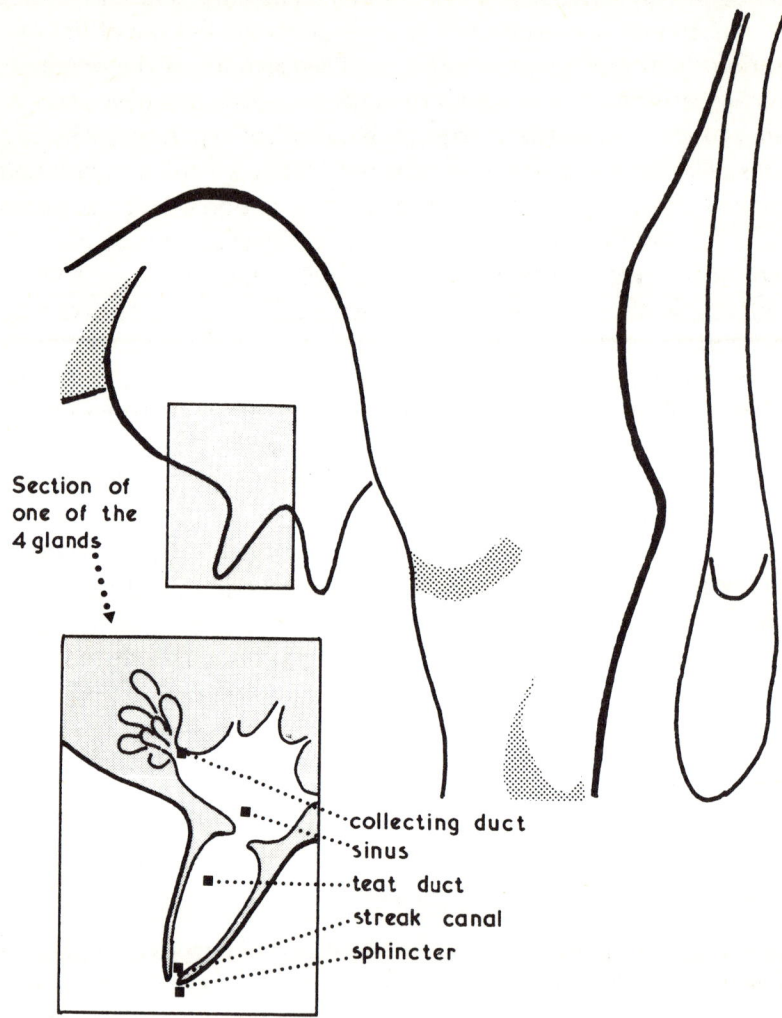

Section of
one of the
4 glands

····collecting duct
··sinus
····teat duct
···streak canal
···sphincter

Figure 25

The period of decline of sexual activity after oestrus, occurring at the same time as the decline of the corpus luteum is known as *di-oestrus* in the cow and *metoestrus* in the bitch, di-oestrus being a short period between oestrous cycles, while metoestrus is the period before complete sexual activity or *anoestrus*, such as one finds in the bitch.

The male hormones

In the male, sexual hormones are responsible for the build-up of male characteristics including size and muscular development. These substances are known as *androgens*, and some are available commercially. *Testosterone* is commonly used, sometimes in the control of the female cycle, and other synthetic androgens have been used to stimulate beef production in steers.

Drugs used to influence the sexual cycle

The control of the natural sexual cycle is achieved by a delicate balance of hormones, at different stages one becoming dominant over the other. Because the effects of sexual hormones are so profound, considerable research has been carried out to see whether the cycle may be influenced to make the animals more productive, or merely more convenient for man to keep. Four basic commercially available hormones are required in order to regulate the cycle by artificial means.

The female hormones or oestrogens—These are available as stilboestrol, either in tablets for implantation or in solution for injection.

The pregnancy hormones or progestagens—Several potent substances are available for use sometimes by mouth and sometimes by injection. Megestrol acetate is an example of the former, and methroxyprogesterone an example of the latter.

Chorionic gonadotrophin or luteinizing hormone (LH) is obtained from the urine of women in early pregnancy.

Serum gonadotrophin or follicle stimulating hormone (FSH) is obtained from the blood of mares in early pregnancy.

THE ENDOCRINE SYSTEM

Certain organs such as the liver, the salivary glands and the seminal vesicles pour their secretions out into the body through special ducts. However, there is another system of organs called the endocrine organs which pour their secretions directly into the blood stream. These secretions are called 'hormones'. They play an important part in regulating the chemistry of the body and so can be described as 'chemical messengers'. Some glands produce two secretions, one of which is released through a duct and the other, a hormone, is discharged into the circulation.

The pancreas

The pancreas, as we have seen, produces digestive juices or enzymes, but it also produces a hormone called *insulin*. Insulin makes it possible for the liver to store glycogen or starch. Without insulin the liver would be unable to store glycogen and this would be poured into the blood stream as sugar causing a disease called diabetes, which simply means too much sugar in the blood. When this disease occurs, the patient is given injections of insulin.

The thyroid

Placed on the side of the trachea, the thyroid produces a 'growth hormone'. Without this hormone the body does not grow properly and mental deficiency results.

The adrenals

The adrenals are small organs lying (in cattle) in front of each kidney, and they are vital to the maintainence of life. They consist of two parts, an outer layer, known as the cortex, and an inner or medullary layer. The medullary layer is responsible for the production of *adrenaline* which is a hormone which prepares the body to make a supreme temporary effort. Such an effort might be required for instance when an animal has to run away from a lion or other predator. In general, adrenaline strengthens the heart beat and restricts the amount of blood reaching those tissues which are not required to combat the emergency, it therefore has the effect of concentrating the blood supply and the excess oxygen required in the brain and the muscles.

The cortex produces a substance with a very complex function, and known as a corticosteroid. Its effects are discussed in Section V but again in general it is responsible for regulating the metabolism of the body. This is done in part by seeing that the body fluids are neither too acid nor too alkaline in reaction.

The pituitary

This is the most important ductless gland in the body and lies just under the brain with which it connects. Many of the hormones it releases into the blood stream are increased or decreased in accordance with messages about the outside of the body sent by way of the senses, that is sight, smell, taste, hearing, touch and general comfort and discomfort.

The most important function is the control of the female reproductive cycle. This is explained in detail elsewhere but it is important to realise that the sexual cycle is regulated by the pituitary gland, and that the pituitary gland is regulated by messages from the brain.

The ovaries and testicles

These organs also produce hormones, and again their relationship with the sexual cycle is explained elsewhere; here it is only necessary to make two points. Female hormone or oestrogen is responsible for feminine appearance as well as those changes in the female sexual organs associated with reproduction. Male hormone or androgen is responsible for masculine attributes such as muscular development and aggressive behaviour.

THE ANATOMY AND PHYSIOLOGY OF THE CHICKEN

Birds differ very considerably from mammals and it is necessary to consider these differences very carefully since they affect the standards by which the health of chicken are judged, and the types of diseases from which they suffer.

The skeleton

The axial skeleton consists of the skull, vertebral column, the ribs and the sternum.

The skull

The obvious difference from mammals is the beak which is without

THE SKELETON OF THE CHICKEN

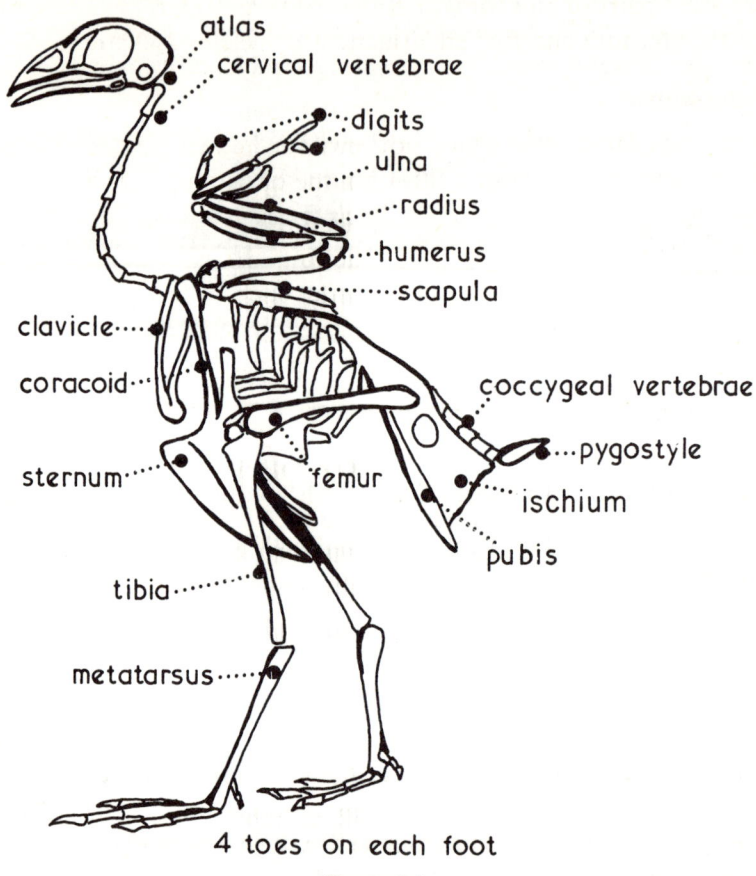

4 toes on each foot

Figure 26

teeth, and the two large sockets which in life carry the eyes.   The brain cavity in birds is notoriously small.

The vertebral column

There are 14 cervical or neck vertebrae in birds and they allow for a long sinuous neck.   The vertebrae in the lumbar sacral region are fused into a bony mass consisting of 16 vertebrae.   This is the platform which carries the legs, and in the chicken the legs are very well

developed since it is a ground dweller.   There are 6 coccygeal vertebrae in the tail.

The ribs

There are 7 pairs of ribs, of which two pairs are floating and do not
reach the sternum and five are attached to the ribs and sternum.

The sternum

This is a very large bone which not only forms a foundation for the
powerful wing muscles but a floor for the chest and a great part of the
abdomen.

The wings

These take the place of arms in the mammal and, while they are specially adapted, the same bones are recognizable.

The hindlegs

These again are adapted to the life style of birds but the bones are
recognizably similar to those of mammals and bear the same names.

The digestive system

The process of preparing food for digestion differs very considerably
from that of mammals.   The beak allows of food being seized and
swallowed but never chewed.   It is probable that birds do not taste
food in the way that mammals do.   The food is taken into the oesophagus which has a large swelling just in front of the chest known as
the crop.   From the crop the digestive tract enters the glandular part
of a very muscular organ known as the gizzard.   It is here that the
food is ground up by means of pieces of stone which have been
swallowed and held in the gizzard for this purpose.   The gizzard
opens into a small intestine consisting of a duodenum, jejunum, and
an ileum just as in mammals.   The large intestine consists of the caeca
and the colon.   The caeca are two blind tubes which are about 18 cm
(7 in) long in the fowl, and which empty into the intestine where the
ileum joins the colon.   They provide a large area of cells from which
absorption of food substances can take place.

The colon empties into the cloaca which is the common opening
for the digestive, urinary and genital systems.   The liver is a large

structure in birds which occupies a large part of the abdominal cavity in front of the gizzard.

The pancreas is also easily seen; it is a narrow gland lying between loops of the small intestine.   The spleen is a rounded reddish brown body.

The respiratory system

The nostrils are found at the top of the beak and lead into the pharynx and from there into the trachea which leads into the rather small lungs.   Birds have developed a respiratory system dependent on air sacs which are found in the body cavity as well as in the long axis of the large limb bones.   In principle, the air moves through the lungs into the air sacs and is presented with a large area for the absorption of oxygen and the expiration of carbon dioxide.

The urogenital system

The kidneys lie on each side of the vertebral column and are very fragile; they bear little resemblance to mammalian kidneys.   The ureters carry the urine from the kidneys to the cloaca where it is voided through the vent with the contents of the colon.

The testicles of the cock vary in size in accordance with the season, as most birds are very seasonal in their reproductive patterns. They are found in the abdomen and are bean-shaped and yellowish in colour.   The ductus deferens opens up on to a small papillae lying in the cloaca.

The ovaries of the hen start off as two in number but the right one rapidly disappears during development of the chick and it is the left one which enlarges and is responsible for producing the eggs.   The ova consist of yolk only when leaving the ovary and passing into the oviduct, the egg white is added some half way down the tube, and the egg shell just before the oviduct enters the cloaca and before it is laid through the vent.   The egg shell is soft when the egg is first laid but hardens as it meets the outside air.

The circulatory system

The heart is similar to that found in mammals in that it has four

REPRODUCTION IN BIRDS

THE EGG

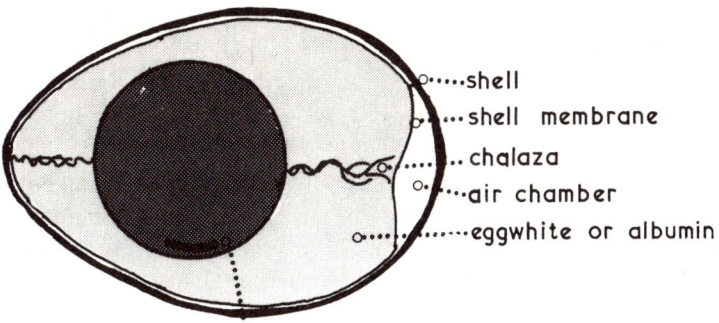

·····shell

···shell membrane

··chalaza

·air chamber

······eggwhite or albumin

germinal disk at edge of eggyolk

THE REPRODUCTIVE TRACT

ova in left ovary·······
(the right ovary is not
formed in birds)

the yolk & germinal disk are
formed in ovary & pass
into the infundibulum·

the eggwhite is added in
the oviduct & ampulla····

the membrane & shell are
added in the isthmus··

uterus ·········

rectum ············   ureter

egg in soft shell laid from
cloaca ···

Figure 27

chambers, the right and left auricles and the right and left ventricles. The circulation is much the same in principle but differs considerably in detail. Blood corpuscles in chickens are nucleated so may be easily distinguished from those of mammals.

THE THEME OF THIS SECTION

The opportunity is taken to emphasize the following points:

(1) The body is composed of cells, divided between organs. Some cells are specialized in their function, but many more are found as the 'building blocks' in all organs and parts of the body.

(2) The skeleton is the framework on which the body rests, and the voluntary muscles act by contracting and drawing two bones together across a joint. Involuntary muscles are found as part of tissues and provide them with the movement they need to fulfil their functions.

(3) The body is dependent on water to survive, and the circulatory system exists to carry substances in solution or suspension to all parts of the body.

(4) The digestive canal surrounds food substances lying outside the body, in that substances contained within it are separated from the body tissues by the *epithelial* lining of the intestine.

(5) The respiratory system is open to the environment, and the delicate cells in the air sacs have to be protected from foreign substances present in the air.

(6) A study of blood and urine provides a useful means of assessing the health of the animal.

(7) The body is regulated in two ways. By conscious effort through the nervous system, or unconscious effort through nervous reflexes, and secondly by chemical regulation largely by hormones.

(8) The body is only studied as a series of separate systems for convenience. No system or organ functions in isolation, each one is interdependent with the others, and disease in one produces effects in other organs, and in the ability of the body to survive, to grow, and to reproduce.

Section II

Animal Behaviour

INTRODUCTION AND GENERAL COMMENTS

The behaviour of animals is directly related to the chosen method of survival. The most obvious behaviour patterns are clearly species specific, and have been developed by inheritance. Thus the highly specialized behaviour required in order to seek out and consume vegetable matter is totally different from that of a carnivore which seeks other animals as food. It might be true to say that the way of life, and association between animals of the same species, is governed by their need to eat.

The broad patterns of behaviour are clear to see, but there are variations on the main theme that repay close study. A knowledge of the innate response of a domestic animal to a series of stimuli can make farm work very much easier. To mention but one simple example: cows move into a milking parlour in a definite order when left to themselves and in the absence of strangers. A completely unknown milkman can reduce the milk yield considerably merely by altering the order in which he carries out his duties from that of his predecessor, and by altering the order in which the animals enter their stalls.

One can hardly discuss behaviour without bringing into consideration the attitude that veterinary workers ought to display to the animals under their care. It helps to consider several aspects, some of them over-publicized, which influence the way in which one regards animals.

The exploitation of animals

This highly emotive word in the title of this paragraph is used advisedly.   There has never been a time when man could exist in the absence of animals, and there is no likelihood that he will be called upon to do so in the foreseeable future.   It is quite impossible to return to some quite fictional time in the distant past when man was in balance with 'nature'.   Man has always exploited those animals which he could rear and use, but to say this is not to absolve him of the responsibility that such actions imply.   It makes sound commercial sense to keep animals in contentment although it is impossible for any human being to define what an animal might regard as luxury.   The need is therefore to keep the animals without stress in the most efficient way possible.

There is also no possibility that man will give up his mechanical implements, nor that he will be able to make meaningful decreases in his food demands on animal.   The pattern is towards intensive production; and it is necessary to make quite sure that we so understand natural behaviour patterns of each domestic species that we may accomplish this in a way which will cause the minimum of distress. The greatest stress is provided by disease, and successful prevention and control of disease is most likely to follow careful application of animal husbandry methods worked out in cooperation with the specialist in behaviour.

Intelligence in animals

The chicken behaves like an animated automaton.   It responds automatically and without thought, for instance, by running away from an overhead shadow.   Chickens retain only a vestige of individual choice of behaviour.   Herbivores are less intelligent than carnivores but they can learn to avoid danger and to seek fresh food or water; they give the impression however, of being less flexible than carnivores in responding to unforeseen hazards.   Carnivores clearly must retain some ability to innovate because chasing prey is not a mechanical process.   Hyenas have been shown, for instance, to spell each other in following gazelle, and to cut across the diameter of a circle that the fleeing animal is pursuing.   It is also apparent that carnivores can usually be taught far more circus routines than can herbivores.   The sole exception is the horse which responds with unthinking confidence to human signals.

The attitude of man to animals

It is clear that many human beings have great sympathy for animals, but it is also clear that this sympathy is more obvious when the person concerned is not in a survival trap.   Primitive people who depend for their existence on the vagaries of weather, and who are too poor to store any quantity of food, are far less sentimental in their contacts with animals.   They behave very much as animals do, they live from day to day, and except in very simple terms do not try to look forward into what can only be an uncertain future.   To survive to the next sunrise is sufficient objective in life; naturally this is associated with a close family or tribal structure since cooperation is a means to survival.

It seems apparent from behavioural study that animals live even more concentrated lives.   They have little means of comparison, they cannot regret that which they have never had.   The philosophy of animal management would appear therefore to hinge on two things.   Animals should be kept with the minimum of physical discomfort and in surroundings which cause them no distress.   Their ailments should be dealt with promptly, and when they come to the time of their death, they should be destroyed without pain and without consciousness of danger.

These requirements can be met within the compass of commercial exploitation.   The details are a matter of judgement, but a close and scientific investigation of the behaviour of each animal species must make possible the achievement of these ideals, with profit to the farmer, and within the conscience of man.

The necessity for restraint of animals

The following pages mention only the more obvious points in regard to animal behaviour, and the subject may be further studied in the books listed in the appendix, but every animal worker is well advised to observe animals and form his own opinions.

The area which he is obliged to study is the behaviour of animals under restraint.   All animals restrained for treatment behave as

though they are in great danger.   The fable of the lion which asked
for the thorn to be taken out of its foot, and then accepted an obli-
gation to its helper, has perpetuated a fallacy.   Animals resent
handling unless they have been taught otherwise.   When they allow
it they do so because they have learnt that it is pleasurable.   The
astonishment of a sheltered pet injected, and therefore hurt for its
own good, has only to be seen for this truism to be realized.   It is
impossible to explain anything to an animal.

The handler must therefore learn to read the danger response
signals of each species.   If any animal is to be hurt for more than a
moment then anaesthesia or tranquilization ought to be considered.
This is not only in the interests of the animal but in those of the
attendants.

Fortunately, most animals signal their intentions ahead of their
actions because the first reflex response to danger is to warn the
aggressor that they mean business.   In bulls it is a swelling of the
neck, a lowering of the head and the pawing of the ground.   In dogs
it is the raising of the lip and the narrowing of the eyes.   Horses
tend to show the whites of their eyes and pigs to grunt.   Cats are by
far the most dangerous because they show little expression before
they demonstrate their displeasure.   It is practically impossible to
hold a thoroughly alarmed cat.

BEHAVIOUR PATTERNS WITHIN EACH SPECIES

Cattle

It has already been mentioned that cattle are of two types; those are
known as *Bos taurus*, which are probably descended from the wild
aurochs of the plains areas of Europe, and *Bos indicus* known as the
'zebu' which is possibly descended from the Malayan banteng, a wild
ox adapted to a tropical climate.   These cattle types differ to some
extent from each other but cattle the world over have certain behaviour patterns in common.   Both types interbreed but most work on
behaviour of bovines comes from research groups in temperate zones.

Feeding behaviour
Cattle stand to graze and differ from horses in the way that they take

grass.   The tongue is used to curl around the bunch of grass stems which are nipped between the incisors and the hard palate on the upper jaw.   The stems are broken by moving the head, and the grass is swallowed without very much chewing.   Cattle appear to prefer to graze in the very early morning and in the late evening, although they will also feed for short periods of time during the day.   Zebu animals cannot hold as much food in their digestive systems as can temperate breeds, and therefore need to move about more than they do and to feed more frequently.   It is for this reason that it is so important that when animals are placed at night in a *khola, boma* or *kraal*, they should be released as soon as possible in the morning. Similarly, they should be replaced in the *boma* as late as possible at night.

Cattle tend to face all in the same direction when grazing, and it is noticeable that zebu cattle keep closer together than do other breeds of cattle.   If they have a choice they choose the herbage that they like; sometimes they only like a species of grass at one stage in its growing cycle.   They are also influenced by weather and prefer to graze when it is cool.

All cattle ruminate; that is they regurgitate the contents of the rumen and chew it over in the mouth by sideways movements of the jaw before reswallowing it.   The food is fermented in the rumen so that the more the grass is cut down and crushed the better it will digest.   Rumination has always been thought of as a pleasurable occupation; certainly all ruminants appear to lie down to chew the cud.   Should anything happen to disturb them, rumination stops immediately and the animal stands up if it is lying.   After feeding, three-quarters of the time occupied is taken up by rumination, and it will be obvious that most of the day is occupied with the process of acquiring food if the cattle are at pasture.   This lack of time to ruminate must be taken into account when work oxen are used, and they must not only be fed concentrates but should have some time to graze.

Drinking

Cattle drink by placing their mouth in the water, leaving their nostrils above water level and by sucking the water into the mouth, swallowing it, and passing it down into the rumen.   They do not have to raise their heads in order to swallow.   Water requirement varies with the

DIFFERENCES BETWEEN BOS TAURUS AND BOS INDICUS OR ZEBU CATTLE

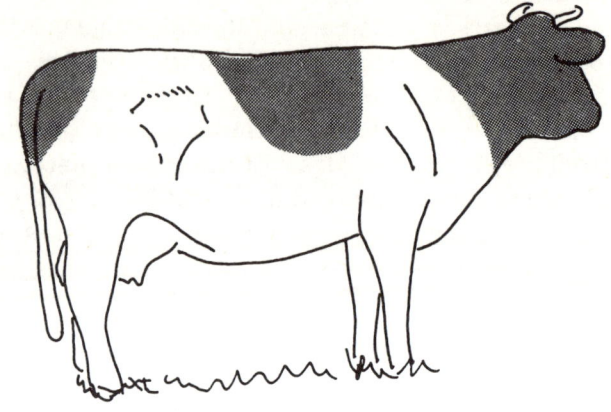

Bos taurus- adapted to a temperate climate and
lush pastures.   It is usually big framed,
matures rapidly & easily separated from its calf.

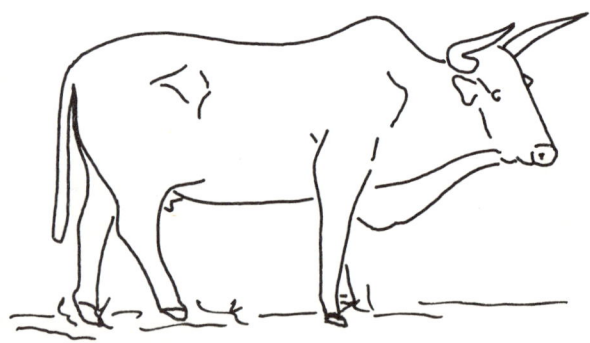

Bos indicus- humped cattle with pronounced dewlaps
adapted to hot dry conditions.

Figure 28

outside temperature and with the type of food, dry and salty food requiring more water than does succulent grazing. The water requirement of zebus is considerably less than that of temperate breeds; in hot arid conditions they need about two-thirds of that required by Herefords, for instance.

Suckling behaviour of calves

The calf begins suckling between 2–5 hours after birth and does so by suction on the teat. It usually stands to suckle with its body lying alongside that of the cow and its tail towards the cow's head. Calves may be taught to drink from buckets, though this requires patience, by dipping fingers in the milk and then placing them in the calf's mouth. It is very important that the calf should be suckled by the cow for the first two or three days of its life, by doing so it acquires the first milk which contains protective substances from the cow which will help to prevent it becoming infected with harmful organisms. Colostrum is an essential food substance for the calf.

Sexual behaviour of cattle

Cattle are gregarious animals; they move about in herds and the males are very different in appearance from the females, the mature male being very much bigger. In the wild state and under range conditions the bulls dominate the females and this factor may be important in successful mating. Cattle form male–female associations only during the act of mating; once this is complete the two sexes drift apart and the bull may then approach another cow.

Natural service

It will be apparent from what has already been said, that in the wild state where one bull accompanies several cows that it is the cow which makes the first move in the reproductive process. The bull is always willing to serve but the cow must first present itself. Because the cow has to seek out the bull a behavioural change occurs when it is coming into heat or oestrus. The first signs are restlessness and a disinclination to feed or to ruminate; it may merely wander round the field aimlessly, occasionally stopping to take a few mouthfuls of grass. This restlessness is also reflected in the milk yield and if this is carefully recorded on a graph at evening and morning milkings, a dip in production will be seen.   Finally, when ovulation is near and oestrus is at its height, the cow will stand for service.   When a bull is present this is the time that the cow is served.

The sexual act is very brief in cattle, although the bull, having detected a cow coming into oestrus, may stay with her for two or three days as heat develops and she becomes more responsive to his presence.   The bull having smelt the vulva of the cow in heat extends its head and makes a distinctive curling of the upper lip.   It next moves alongside and brushes the cow with its head and neck. Finally it mounts and serves within a very short time and slowly dismounts.   Both animals move away and resume their grazing behaviour.

The detection of oestrus in cattle

Few dairy farms nowadays keep a bull because artificial insemination is used to get the cows into calf.   Success depends on the correct timing of the injection of semen.   Clearly, the nearer this happens to the crisis of the oestrus period the better.   This is the point at which the cow will stand to be mounted, and during oestrus the cow in heat will stand to be mounted by other cows, particularly those which in their turn are approaching oestrus.   Another point that is relevant is the fact that heat can sometimes be over quickly in hot weather.   The farmer must therefore, for best results, be able to detect heat as soon as it occurs.   If it is missed, he will have to wait another three weeks before the animal can be served and the total productive life of the cow will be reduced.   Bags of dye are sometimes placed on the backs of cows in the region of the sacrum; when the cow is mounted by others the bag breaks and leaves a red stain which can be seen by the farmer.   Since oestrus often reaches a peak at night this method can be very useful.   Ovulation takes place in the cow some hours after oestrus so that when artificial insemination is used, this must be timed to coincide with ovulation, because sperm does not live more than a few hours in the genital tract.

Artificial insemination

Perhaps it is advisable to say a few words here about artificial insemination in bovines.   AI, as it is called, is possible in this species because of the animals' behavioural pattern.   Bulls readily mount a cow, provided it will stand, and can be induced to ejaculate into a false vagina, even one on a dummy.   The semen is collected, divided into doses, and stored in deep freeze.   When required it is warmed and ejected through special syringes, inserted into the vagina as far as the cervix of the cow.

Leadership in cattle

It is noteworthy that there are differences in the willingness of cattle to lead others.   It is difficult to detect this tendency in grazing patterns, but no doubt careful observation would show that some animals more often lead the way to new pastures than do others.   It is a mistake to think that these leaders are always drawn from the large heavy males; frequently the lead animal is a female and some-times one that is not imposing in size.   Detection of such animals in a herd can help in moving cattle from one pasture to another, into or out of a building or into a crush.   Taking a lead animal first allows the other cattle to follow without fuss.

Other types of behaviour action

Dung is dropped anywhere in the pasture and it does not seem that cattle have any control over the place and time.   They do, however, adopt a typical posture which by arching the back prevents the body from being soiled.   Sick animals or those with diarrhoea do not do this and consequently can be picked out from the herd by the fact that they are soiled.   Females cannot urinate unless they are standing still, but males can and do urinate while they are moving.   The aver-age daily weight of dung voided by zebus is between 9 and 13 kg (19 and 28 lb) per animal depending on the quantity of food ingested.

Calves sleep lying on the brisket with the head resting on the flank, but once rumination has developed at weaning, cattle probably do not lose consciousness.   They may sleep lightly for short periods, but they do not go into deep sleep as do some other species, particu-larly carnivores.

Cattle lick themselves and their companions a great deal during the course of a day, and it is probable that it is in this way that dipped animals absorb arsenic and other dip fluids.   It is also noticeable that animals in poor conditions or suffering from some disease do not lick themselves as frequently; consequently in tick-infested areas, they may be seen to be suffering from a larger tick population than their neighbours.   Such animals should be examined very carefully to try to diagnose the cause of the illness.

Comments on cattle behaviour in general

The remarks made above explain the general behaviour of cattle, in other words what is normally expected of the breed. They cannot attempt to explain the behaviour of each animal as an individual within a herd and in its relationship with human beings. All animals are individuals and each one not only differs in appearance from its neighbours but also differs in its behaviour.

It is the skill of stockmanship to recognize these differences and, by careful observation and by pandering perhaps in small ways to each cow's behaviour pattern, to make the task of management easier. A simple instance is the fact that some animals like to be milked first, others care less about this, and it would be foolish to push an unwilling cow into the milking parlour ahead of a willing one.

It is particularly important for the person doing the milking to know the likes and dislikes of individual cows under his care, since this is the way that early cases of disease and particularly mastitis are detected. Usually the very first indication that something is wrong is a slight variation in behaviour. For instance, a greedy cow may leave part of its food, or a quiet cow may show resentment in being milked.

It is a very good exercise for anyone entering a herd for the first time as a stockman to write down very carefully all the individual characteristics of each cow. Start with the appearance and move on to note its behaviour. The next step is to think one ahead of the cow by working out how one can use this information to make the work of looking after the animal easier and more interesting.

Sheep and goats

Domestic sheep are thought to have originated from wild sheep captured in the eastern Mediterranean, many centuries before the earliest recorded civilizations of that area. Domestic sheep differ from wild sheep in that they have a long tail and it is therefore possible to distinguish their skeletons from those of their wild relatives. In addition, their coats are either of wool or hair but do not contain the two together as found in wild species. It is not possible to tell by examining the skeletal remains of goats whether they are from domesticated or wild species. Wild goats do, however, tend to have thicker horn cores. They too, are thought to have been domesticated in the eastern Mediterranean, probably before sheep.

Feeding behaviour

Sheep have a split upper lip and graze in a different way from cattle. They cut off the grass between the bottom incisors and the hard pad which replaces the incisors in the upper jaw; the tongue is not used in this process. This is an important difference in disease diagnosis since sheep with tongue lesions will still feed when infected with foot-and-mouth disease while cattle will not. The primary sign of this condition in sheep is tenderness in walking. Grass grazed by sheep is cut off nearer the ground than is the case with cattle.

Goats are browsers rather than grazers; that is they prefer twigs and leaves of trees, and will strip bark if they cannot reach the branches. It is thought that this habit has been responsible for killing many of the trees in areas where goats were first kept in large numbers such as the eastern Mediterranean. Goats can withstand a high degree of bitterness and even appear to prefer bitter-tasting branches or vegetation.

The most concentrated grazing of sheep takes place in daylight hours starting at sunrise and continuing in short periods throughout the day with periods of rest and lying down to ruminate. They rarely graze at night. Sheep move about the grazing in groups facing in the same direction; goats tend to disperse more widely and, particularly when grazing among shrubs, seem to keep together more by hearing, or perhaps by smelling, their neighbours than by seeing them.

Sexual behaviour

In the temperate zones sheep have a well marked breeding season. This is less pronounced near the equator and breeding may take place at all times of the year in consistently hot countries. The males are intensely active at the time that the ewes come into oestrus and may serve up to 15 ewes a day. Female sheep start to come into heat in the temperate areas when the days get shorter in late autumn, with peak oestrus around the shortest day, and the oestrus cycles last on average 18 days if the ewe does not become pregnant. The goat behaves in a similar way; in the temperate areas it comes into season in the autumn, heat periods are said to last rather longer than in the ewe, the length of the oestrous cycle being about 21 days.

Other differences between sheep and goats

It would seem by observation that goats have been less domesticated by breeding than is the case with sheep. Goats climb more and will leave their kids while they seek out food; the kids retain the ability to freeze when something alarms them. In similar circumstances sheep and lambs react by joining the flock and then by moving off in a close bunch; goats move away in a much more loosely bunched group, much as their wild relatives do. Consequently, it is easier to herd sheep with a dog. Sheep are easily driven but goats are better led.

Disease resistance

It is noticeable that goats are more resistant to disease than sheep, and they seem more resistant to adverse conditions. This may be because they commonly feed on herbage which has not been contaminated with dung and is more likely to be free from internal parasites.

Pigs

Pigs are interesting animals since they have proved to be very adaptable both in domestication and in the wild. The sows have large litters and their ability to eat all kinds of food means that they can be intensively fed in comparatively large units with mixtures of protein, fat and carbohydrates. They are also quick growing and the sows may be served again shortly after weaning the piglets.

Feeding behaviour

The consistency of the food supplied to pigs does not appear to influence their uptake; they will readily take dry meal or pellets and are fond of animal matter such as earthworms and even small mammals. They have a well defined sense of smell and will readily seek out food by rooting in ground which they search with their snouts. They can be persuaded to eat solid food within a few days of birth and appear to eat more when there is competition to reach the food trough. In other words, pigs reared in isolation do not eat so well as those reared together. Pigs like to drink and eat in succession, they eat a little and drink a little until satisfied.

Sexual behaviour

In the wild the boar is dominant and herds his sow and litter as they move about looking for food. The boar and sow do not part after service and may remain together for considerable periods of time. Domesticated pigs appear to have some traces of this behaviour since some boars appear to prefer some sows, but normally the boars breed readily. Oestrus lasts 1–5 days and the time between cycles is roughly 21 days. Oestrous cycles continue until the sow becomes pregnant, and the sow will come into oestrus again about 9 days after the piglets have been weaned. The gestation period is 113–116 days.

Other behaviour of interest

Pigs are intensely curious and it is obviously calming to them if they are bedded on straw or similar material that they can root about. An alternative is to give them an old tyre to play with. It is possible that some of the vices they acquire in intensively kept units, such as tail-biting, are due to boredom. They will, if their pens permit, use one place to dung and urinate. They like to wallow and should be sprayed with water in hot weather.

Dogs

The behaviour of dogs has been discussed and investigated on all planes from the extreme scientific to the extreme emotional, and it is therefore difficult to establish a clear concensus of opinion about basic interpretation. Dogs were probably the first domesticated animal; archeological findings show that dogs were present in neolithic settlements over 8000 years ago, and even today primitive human communities often have no domesticated animal other than the dog. This long history and the constant selection by breeding for a number of work requirements probably accounts for the great number of different breeds found throughout the world.

The dog is a carnivore and in the wild state lives in packs. Carnivores tend to be much more intelligent than herbivores, probably because a certain intelligence is required to seek out and kill other animals. It is the necessity for wild canines, which have to work as a pack, to defer to their pack leader, and above all to learn to co-ordinate hunting approaches which makes the dog so useful to man.

Feeding patterns

Wild dogs are used to eating in quantity when food is available and doing without it when it is not.   As a result, dogs eat food rapidly, seizing it and gulping until it is finished.   This process is speeded up in the presence of another dog and potential competitor for the food.   It is for this reason that pet dogs should be fed once a day, except for pregnant bitches which may not be able to eat sufficient food to meet their needs in one meal.

Sexual and reproductive behaviour

The dog is quite unique among domesticated animals in that the bitch only has one reproductive cycle in its heat period.   In the wild state the bitch comes into heat only once a year, although domesticated dogs usually have two periods a year.   At each heat there is a prolonged and intensive cycle.   It is therefore important to the species that the chances of breeding successfully should be enhanced at that time.   It is very noticeable that the male dog is far more interested in a bitch coming into heat, and at an earlier stage in the cycle, than is the case in other animals.   Similarly, the bitch actively seeks out the dog at this time, and when mating does take place, it is a very prolonged process. Mechanically, the dog becomes 'tied' into the female early in copulation; this is clearly a mechanism to improve the chances of conception.   The bulb of the penis swells and becomes lodged in the vagina of the female, and ejaculation takes place over several minutes in conditions which make the passage of the sperms towards the ova that much less hazardous than is the case in other animals.   This is a wonderful adaptation to improve the chances of conception, since in the wild state a failure could mean the bitch having no chance of reproduction for a further year.

There is another very interesting adaptive procedure to ensure survival of the pups.   Bitches which do not become pregnant after heat frequently suffer from what is called false pregnancy.   This occurs about six weeks after heat.   They go through all the motions of making a bed, and mammary development and secretion.   Clearly, while this is a disadvantage to owners, it must enable orphaned puppies in a pack to be reared by barren bitches.

Other characteristics

The in-built survival mechanism of the wild dog involves co operation within the pack.   It must learn quickly to follow the patterns of behaviour of its companions in order to survive.   Man makes use of this characteristic in regulating his association with the animal. Successful control of dogs involves mastership over them, just as hierarchical organization is rapidly established for a new member of the pack.   A dog entering a pack quickly learns who it may command and who it must obey.   Similarly in relationships with human beings, a dog which is not mastered will attempt to dominate, and it ought to be accepted that there must exist dogs which cannot be mastered by anyone.   Such animals are very rare, but they have no future in a human society.

It is a common saying that you cannot teach an old dog new tricks, and in general this is very true.   All the evidence suggests that a dog is happiest when it learns its place in youth, and when conditions continue to be as they were when it was first taught its place in its household.   Confusion in dogs arises when they have no clear indication of where they fit into human society, in other words who is the pack leader, and when having established a pack leader, that leader changes with a change of ownership.

Dogs are easily trained not to defaecate and urinate in the house; this is because they are already conditioned to this pattern of behaviour.   However, a dog under extreme stress, that is in a state of nervous excitement, will automatically defaecate and urinate no matter where it is.   This is a natural release mechanism so that the animal is not impeded in making a maximum effort of survival.   It is quite useless to punish an animal for doing this; by punishment one is reinforcing the mechanism, and making it more likely that it will do it perhaps more readily the next time it is upset.

Another point of interest is that dogs communicate with each other by means of barks, facial movements of the lips and eyebrows, and movements of the body and tail.   Each individual dog develops slight variations in the way it does this.   The domesticated dog uses these same means in trying to communicate with human beings, and it is worth studying dogs as individuals to see what they mean by their behaviour patterns.   There is little doubt that the most successful dog handlers automatically register the messages given out by their charges and act upon them.

Summary

The dog is the oldest, and arguably, the most important domestic animal. Should man ever become completely mechanized, then it is possible that the dog will be the only domestic animal to survive the process. The value of the dog is in its adaptability, and the ease with which it can form a workable relationship with man. To say this is not to be sentimental; it is hard fact that more human beings have contact with dogs than with any other domesticated animal. No person seeking to work with animals can ignore this. Dogs are part of human life and as such are deserving of careful scientific study.

Horses

The horse is a very curious animal, since it does not fit into any precise pattern. It is a herbivore but its digestive system appears less specialized in turning vegetable matter into digestive substances than the ruminant. Its stomach is simple although the intestine is heavily modified to deal with the great quantities of roughage which it needs to digest. Wild horses have to be trained to eat concentrated food, and those types of horse which have been most successfully developed by man for specialized functions tend to be those which will take concentrated foods most readily.

The animal's greatest specialization is the development of its legs to achieve the maximum possible speed; not only have these been modified anatomically by the great extension of the bones of one toe on each leg, but the muscles of the legs and back are so arranged that the animal can produce a great width of stride at each thrust. The mechanical effect is to push the horse through the air by means of powerful spaced piston-like thrusts of each leg driven against the ground in succession. Naturally, the legs take an enormous strain and hence the saying that 'a horse is only as good as its legs'.

Feeding behaviour

The horse uses its very strong and mobile lips to draw grass between its two pairs of incisor teeth so that it may be nipped off. It grazes one or two mouthfuls, lifts its head and grinds the grass between its molars and it walks forward a pace, swallows and bends its head down to the grass again. It will not eat grass soiled with its faeces.

Because the horse's teeth are modified to crush grass into comparatively small sections it would appear to be less able to crush grains when they are presented as concentrates. As has been mentioned, the stomach is simple and the boluses of food are rapidly passed through it into the intestine. If too much grain is eaten, this may swell in the stomach and can cause serious distention and pain.

Sexual and reproductive behaviour

The mare is seasonally polyoestrous; this means that there are several cycles of roughly three weeks duration concentrated around the spring equinox in the northern hemisphere. By convention in the United Kingdom, all thoroughbreds (animals used for racing) are deemed to be one year older on each 1 January. It follows therefore that if a foal is born on 2 January it will be one year old on the following January, but one born on 31 December, will be two years old. Since the most lucrative races are for two-year-olds and three-year-olds, the nearer foaling can be arranged to the right side of January each year, the more valuable the animal. In practice, the spacing is one of degree since few mares will breed readily until at least the end of February, and the gestation period of the mare is eleven months. Nevertheless, an extra month of maturity can be very important in two-year-old races.

In the wild, stallions will herd a number of mares in the breeding season, serving them as they come on heat; but in domestication, only selected stallions are kept, and each one is so valuable that it is led up to a mare known to be in oestrus.

The courtship routine, while brief, is perhaps a little more prolonged than in the bovine, but the stallion will serve a mare readily, and the mare will stand to service if oestrus is present.

Other behaviour characteristics

Horses are very aware of slight stimuli from their riders and can be trained to respond to small changes of signal. They are very positive in their response, and they will pick up an undesirable trait as quickly as a desirable one. Thus, having been given the signal the horse in training should be guided into the response; it should not under any circumstances be given a choice of what it might do.   Even in trained horses, confused signals lead to confused horses, and it is for this reason that spirited animals are so hard for inexperienced riders to manage.

The horse is geared to rapid flight from danger, and its eyes are placed so that it has a good view to the side and backwards.   Anything following causes the novice horse great alarm, and horses have to be trained to accept the presence of a carriage or a cart pulled behind them.   Even so, the automatic response of a frightened horse is to gallop away from the danger; this produced many an accident through bolting in the days when horses were the main motive force for transport.

Horses kick in two ways.   The most violent is by balancing on the fore hooves and kicking back with both hinds; to do this they must lower the head to achieve the right centre of gravity.   This is a fighting manoeuvre adapted to enable two stallions to compete for mares. The other kick is a side kick and more often arises from irritation, or of course it can be learnt as a vice.

Intelligence is difficult to assess in horses, mainly because they are so responsive to signals.   Jumping, for instance, is not a natural behaviour and horses show little tendency to jump out of a field even when pressed into a gallop of alarm, but probably all show-jumping is possible because the horse can respond to signals from the rider indicating when to take off.   The convention of horse and rider acting as one is not an idle statement, the value of the horse to man arises from its ability to do what is required of it quickly and with unthinking confidence in its master.   No intelligent animal would carry another mammal on its back into a cavalry charge, but many horses carried their riders to their own certain deaths in the Napoleonic wars.

Stable vices

Horses confined for long periods in stables often develop vices.   They will, for instance, seize a piece of the woodwork in their mouths and swallow air.   Sometimes too, they develop a habit of weaving from side to side.   A similar characteristic is seen in zoo animals kept in cages.   It is probable that normally active animals have a positive stimulus to constant muscular movement.

Cats

Cats were probably domesticated shortly after man started to cultiv-
ate cereals in the fertile crescent of the Middle East.   One may specu-
late that this arose from the necessity to protect the granaries from
small rodents.   Cats were already established in houses in Egyptian
times.

They are not so diverse in their breeds as are dogs, and this may be
because they have not been bred to improve their function.   From
ancient times cats were encouraged to destroy rodents which might
otherwise destroy food crops; gradually, and possibly because they
followed mice into houses, they became established as human companions.   While the appearance of cats has been altered by selective
breeding, there has been no attempt to alter the behavioural patterns.

Cats are obligatory carnivores, that is they are organized to stalking
and killing prey without assistance from companions.   For this reason
they have fewer means of communication with their fellows other
than signs which denote aggressive protection of hunting territory,
such as the raising of the fur and the lashing of the tail.   The necessity to seek out edible prey appears also to have made them intensely
curious, they will respond to any small movement and investigate it.

Feeding patterns

Cats like to take their prey into a corner and to eat it carefully.   They
are delicate feeders easily disturbed.   They do not react to competition because in the natural state they eat alone.   They do, however,
have very large stomachs and can ingest a large meal at one time;
again in the natural state an animal will eat to capacity where it can,
and perhaps go several days until the next meal.

Sexual and reproductive behaviour

The sexual behaviour of the cat is well adapted to ensuring that the
species reproduces itself despite the fact that they are solitary animals.
The female is seasonally polyoestral, that is it comes into heat at
certain seasons of the year, and while in heat there are several cycles
if it is not mated.   Normally the breeding seasons in temperate
regions occur between late January and early March and again in
May and June.   There is a period of anoestrus or absence of sexual

activity between September and early January. However, this cycle varies in various parts of the world probably as daylight varies.

The adaptive behaviour consists of the fact that it is the female or queen which calls when in season, and the male or tom which is attracted. Ovulation only takes place at coitus, so improving the chances of a conception.

Other characteristics

Cats in the wild seek out a resting place and hunt around it, seldom moving away from the immediate locality except to breed and perhaps under extreme duress to hunt. Domesticated cats are notoriously difficult to move from one house to another. Because they are solitary animals they do not associate home with people, but with buildings. They also lack facial expression, they will growl in anger but rarely snarl, and while they communicate by calling, they would appear to have only three easily recognizable changes of voice. One is the call of the female in heat, one is the call after a successful hunt, and the last an infantile call denoting a wish for food.

Hunting instincts in cats

While domesticated cats frequently retain all their hunting abilities and will respond readily to the jerky movements of small rodents or birds, it is noticeable that often they do not associate hunting and feeding. A cat cannot be expected to feed itself from the results of hunting; food must also be provided if it is to be kept in health.

Chickens

The immediate impression given in watching the activities of any bird, and particularly a chicken, is that it is considerably more mechanistic than is the case with a mammal. One can imagine a computer behaving very much as a chicken does, if it were properly programmed and could be contained in a chicken's brainbox. There seem to be a number of quite mechanical responses to certain situations; and while of course like all living animals, each bird is not exactly similar to its fellow, the variations from usual behaviour seem that much more restricted. This factor has long been recognized by the expression 'chicken brained' meaning unintelligent and unthinking response to circumstances.

Man has however benefited very considerably from these traits.

Feeding behaviour

Chickens will eat a wide variety of types of food, from powders to pellets, and they can therefore be given carefully assessed diets, suitable to the type of production required of them. Thus, there are chick diets high in protein, growing diets suited to the rapid growth of broiler birds, and laying diets which give the hens the food substances that they require to produce large quantities of eggs.

Sexual and reproductive behaviour

By careful genetic selection, man has bred parental care out of laying fowls. This has been relatively easily done because the stimulus to broodiness and the incubation of a number of eggs is in response to heat spots on the breast. These are purely mechanical factors and birds have been selected which do not have them and which therefore will not incubate or brood. On the contrary, they continue to produce eggs until they moult, and this again is a more gradual process than in wild birds and of far less duration. No cock is needed in order to induce the hens to lay eggs; this comes about as the correct age of maturity is reached.

Poultry are easily kept in intensive units and will continue to produce unless some quite extraneous stress such as disease intrudes. It is of interest to note that most modern poultry production depends on the use of vast numbers of hybrid birds, that is, birds whose parent stock in combination produce the right characteristics in their progeny. No broiler or layer can ever be allowed to breed or can be used for commercial breeding since to do so would be to produce birds which vary from their parents in accordance with Mendelian laws.

Other characteristics

It is because birds are so mechanistic in their response that the imprinting that ducklings can be made to show to people and objects present at hatching is so interesting. This would imply that many of the characteristics that man exhibits are not selected by his own choice but are all part of the genetic inheritance. This line of thought leads to profound conclusions which cannot be discussed here. However, those who constantly battle with their conscience about whether chickens should be exploited as they are at present, must take note of the fact that there is a distinct possibility that chickens are not aware of the alternatives. They may merely respond to circumstances, and provided that they have certain basic requirements in regard to stretching space, will readily prosper in crowded surroundings.

Frustration behaviour in chickens

In the natural state hens lay their eggs in nest boxes, one hen to each box. It is possible that the vices of feather picking and cannibalism are related to the failure to find a territory in isolation for laying. Similarly wing flapping and neck stretching are probably natural release mechanisms and frustration habits will appear if the space in which they are kept is insufficient to allow them to do this.

Section III

Animal Production

INTRODUCTION

There is no indication that man can exist without some contact with domestic animals. In sophisticated societies there is a strong preference for high quality meat products, milk and butter still sell well, and the demand for leather has never been so persistent. Despite the presence of synthetic fibres wool still holds its own, although subject to cyclical markets. The inference may be reasonably drawn that the more prosperous man becomes, and the more sophisticated he regards himself to be, the more he treasures the products of animal industry.

In the unsophisticated countries there is no choice; animals are the only economic source of power, they frequently provide essential food elements, and sometimes in their dung fuel for fires. The main problem in communities which would like to move away from poverty, is that they treasure their animals, and keep too many of poor quality. Livestock, and particularly cattle, are the poor man's only bank. For the future of the world, quite apart from that of their own communities, animal owners in such areas have to be persuaded to trade their livestock for cash.

The evidence therefore is that animals are becoming of increasing, not decreasing, importance to the human race. It is the bare bones of how man processes animals and animal products that is discussed in the following pages.

THE PRODUCTION OF FOOD

Meat

Affluent people eat more meat of higher quality; and quality of meat in rich communities is assessed by its tenderness and its taste.   Animals killed when young, and particularly before puberty, are the most tender to eat, but taste in meat develops with age.   Generally speaking, meat from mature animals is tastier but tougher.

Young, tender meat, is expensive because to get the animal heavier at a younger age demands high level of feeding with highly priced food products.   The quality of meat from different parts of the carcass also varies, and again speaking generally, the meat from the hind quarters is considerably more highly valued than that from the forequarters.

A secondary, but no less important, factor is that the more expensive the meat, the more conscious the potential purchasers tend to be of the necessity for careful inspection to make sure that it is not affected with disease.   The significance of this is that when meat is produced in the tropics, it has to comply with the highest standards of meat inspection if the country concerned wishes to export it to the highest priced markets, most of which lie in the temperate climatic areas of the world.

Note that it is quite impossible to produce high quality beef in any quantity from grazing alone.   In order to improve the grazing to the level where it is high producing, a considerable amount of careful grass management is required using relatively expensive fertilizers. Most supplementary food given to animals to produce meat comes from cereal crops which supplement the green plants on which animals graze or browse.

Cattle

Cattle provide most of the meat eaten, both in quantity and value. Beef is sold either as fresh carcasses, which have been chilled for 24–48 hours before sale, or from deep frozen carcasses which have been frozen after chilling.   Carcasses are split down the middle along the line of vertebra into two sides, these are divided again behind the line of the ribs into forequarters and hindquarters.   Carcasses are

PARTS OF A BEEF CARCASE
(names vary with locality)

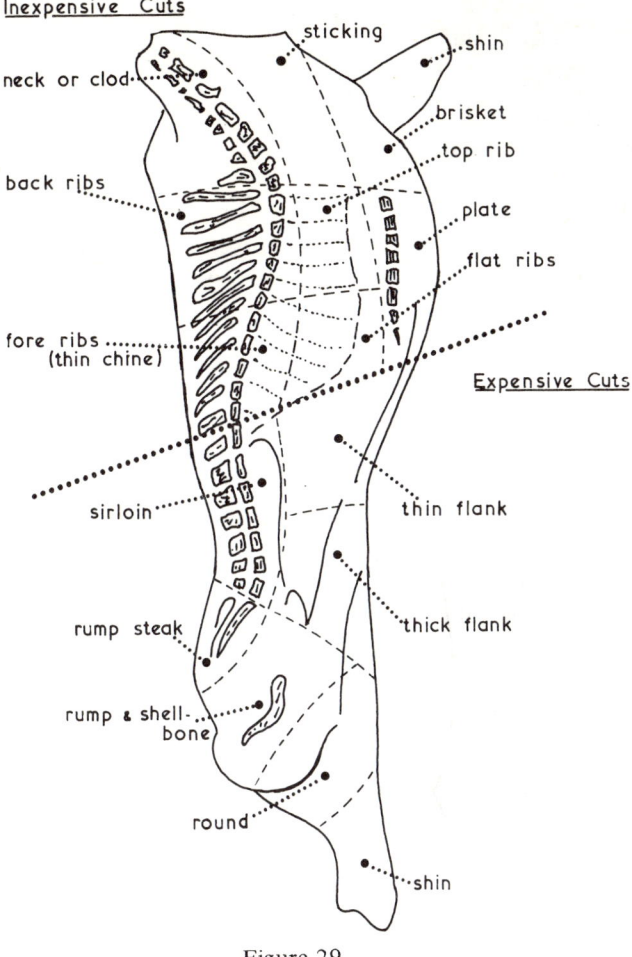

Figure 29

graded by meat graders and sold at prices which vary with grade, young intensively fed animals counting high, and the lowest grade being filled by old animals, many of them off pasture without having received supplementary feeding.

The meat of calves is known as veal.

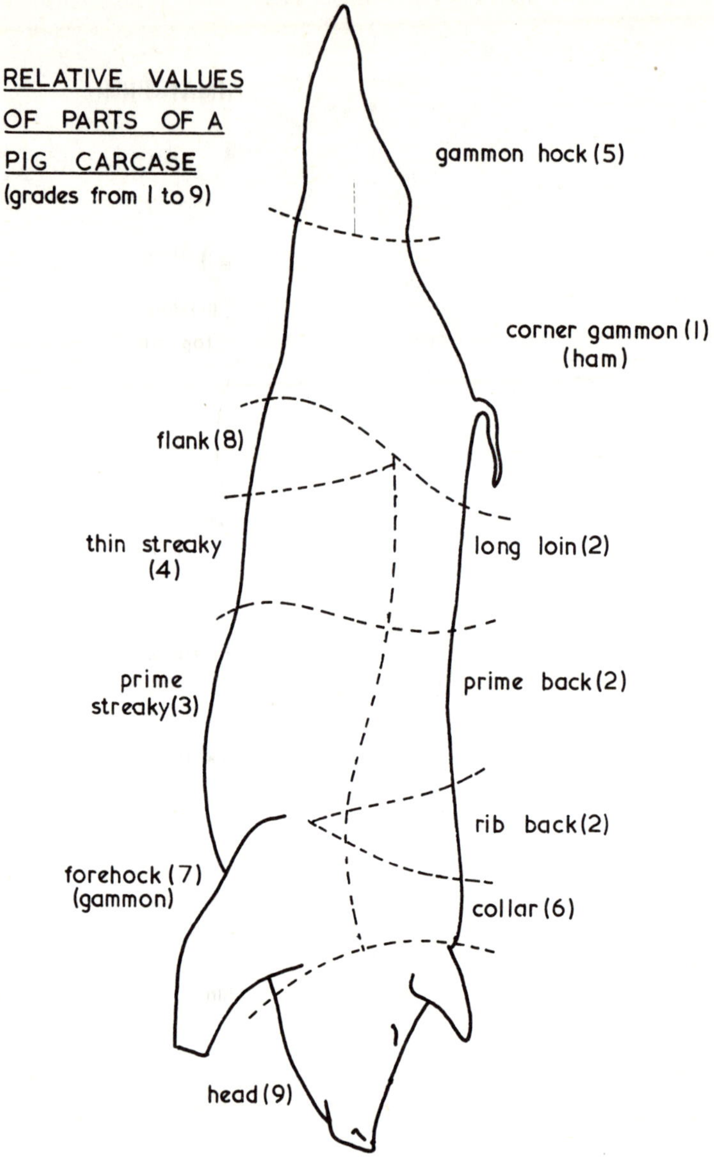

RELATIVE VALUES
OF PARTS OF A
PIG CARCASE
(grades from 1 to 9)

gammon hock (5)

corner gammon (1)
(ham)

flank (8)

thin streaky
(4)

long loin (2)

prime
streaky (3)

prime back (2)

rib back (2)

forehock (7)
(gammon)

collar (6)

head (9)

Figure 30

Pigs

The next most important food animal is the pig. This is because the pig is omnivorous, that is it will eat similar types of food to those eaten by man, it breeds readily (under the best management, twice a year), and large numbers of piglets are produced in each litter. The growth rate of the modern breeds of pig, fed on the right foods in the right proportions, is phenomenal. There are, however, some snags to pig production.

Firstly, pigs eat the same food as man, and the meat they produce is therefore a luxury in so far as most of the human race is concerned. Because it is a luxury, the requirement for pig products fluctuates. When people feel wealthy they buy more of them and when they feel poor, they buy less. The result is that when people start to buy pig meat in quantity there are few pigs and the price rises. As the price rises fewer people can afford to buy pig products, and the farmers are left with the pigs which they have produced to meet the demand but which cannot be sold at the price they have cost to produce. This fluctuation is known as the pig cycle.

The most expensive part of the pig is the hind leg or ham, the next most expensive, the area of the ribs which is made into bacon, and the area of the foreleg which is made into gammon. The other parts of the pig are used in various pig meat products such as pies. Considerably less fresh pork is sold than processed pig meat.

Poultry

Poultry provide the next largest source of meat. Again there is the difficulty of cost of production; vast quantities of poultry are produced in the affluent areas of the world and it provides the most ready source of cheap meat for the mass of the human population. In order to meet this demand, special hybrid birds called 'broilers' have been developed which will reach a weight after a slaughter (dead weight) in the region of 1·5 kg at nine weeks of age. They lack taste but they provide the bulk meat which is so necessary. This is an industry handling millions of birds and the costs of production are such that only a quick throughput can ensure a profit which is often measured in pence per bird slaughtered. This is factory production at its most intensive. The heavier, tastier cockerel, killed at maturity has largely disappeared in Europe. When a larger roasting bird is

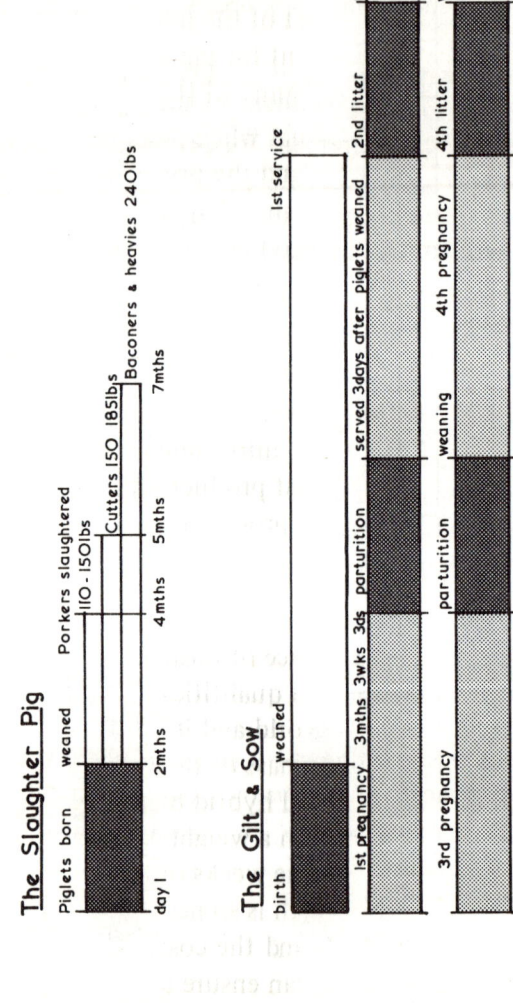

Figure 31

THE LIFE OF THE CHICKEN

All slaughter and laying birds are hybrids — they do not breed true.

The broiler cycle

Eggs from parent stock are incubated and chicks reared in controlled environment houses. Chicken are slaughtered at 1·5–1·75kg liveweight, or 8 to 9 weeks of age.

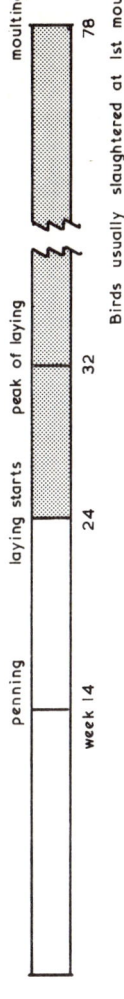

The laying cycle

Day old chicks are sold for rearing as pullets, then placed in cages or houses & known as layers.

Commercial poultry production

Success depends on good food conversion, adequate management & housing but above all careful disease control.

Figure 32

required it is often supplied as a broiler turkey raised under similar conditions with rather greater technical difficulties.

Sheep

No means has yet been devised of producing intensively fed lambs in any quantity. This is because sheep are obligatory grazers and they do not respond to intensive feeding. Furthermore, sheep are seasonal breeders usually only producing at most two lambs a year. They are therefore largely found in those areas of the world which are less densely populated by man but where the grazing is extensive. Because they are such specialized ruminants they also seem to be particularly sensitive to disease, and once the density of sheep in any area is raised above a critical point, trouble in the shape of deaths from disease appears. Because of the pressure of demand for young tender meat, most sheep sold are described as 'lambs'. It is extremely difficult to find mutton, that is meat from older sheep, identified as such on the market.

Rabbits

Other domesticated animals have been farmed as sources of food for man but the only one likely to develop as a source of significance is the rabbit. This animal has many advantages as a meat source; it will feed on cheap products left over from the milling of grain, it breeds regularly and it has large litters, and does not mind crowding. However, it has some disadvantages. Growth rates can be stepped up but taste suffers, and people in some countries are prejudiced against eating rabbits. The biggest drawback is, however, that very much more labour is required to produce rabbits intensively than is the case with poultry, and it is with chicken meat that rabbit meat has to compete in the world market.

Game animals

At the present time the world's meat requirements, as has been seen, are met by two types of domestic animal. Firstly, pigs and poultry

THE SHEEP'S LIFE

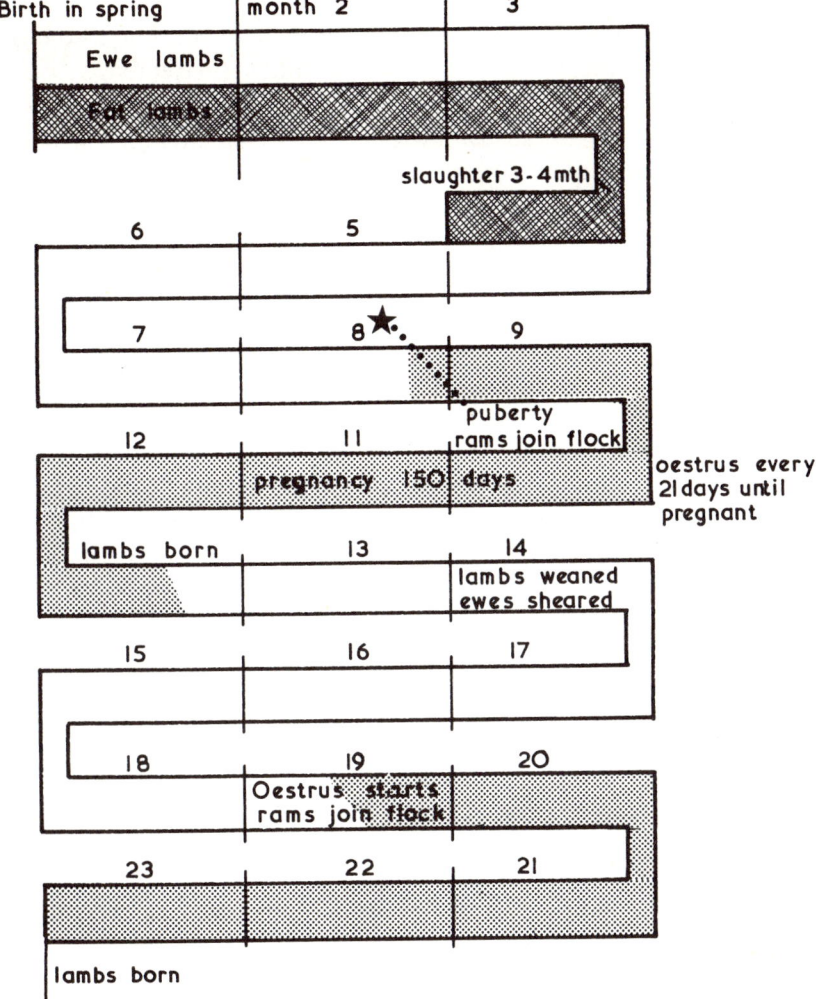

Birth in spring   month 2   3

Ewe lambs

Fat lambs

slaughter 3-4mth

6   5

7   8   9

puberty
rams join flock

12   11
pregnancy 150 days

oestrus every
21 days until
pregnant

lambs born   13   14
lambs weaned
ewes sheared

15   16   17

18   19   20
Oestrus starts
rams join flock

23   22   21

lambs born

Average ewe lives 3-4 years

Figure 33

which are rapid converters of food, and which can be bred in intensive systems capable of turning out great quantities of animals at the right weight and age to meet human tastes.   Secondly, other animals which are able to convert grasses and other vegetation into meat, the rate at which they do this depends on the quality of the grazing and the temperament of the animal.

The characteristics of domestic animals which make them so desirable have been developed over many centuries of selective breeding. No species of game animal has yet been found which is capable of replacing any one of these domestic species.   Game animals which are sold for food usually command high prices, or are bred by rich men for sport.   This is not to say that some species are not of great value in a limited way as food sources, but their limited potential in this respect needs to be recognized.

Fish

While not within the scope of this book, fish are discussed for the sake of completeness.   It should be recognized that they have the advantage of easy breeding, low cost production, rapid growth, and the capability for intensive production that is required of a major human food source.   There is little doubt that fish farming and utilization will increase, and that the control of disease in fish will prove to be as important as the control of disease in mammals.

Milk and eggs

Milk is the most important food obtained from any animal.   It is produced without killing the source of production and the quantity that can be made available from each cow is very great.   It is also the most valuable animal product on the world market, and in the industrialized countries beef animals are usually obtained from the calves produced by milk cows.   It is very difficult to visualize a beef industry in the majority of the countries of the world without a market for milk and milk products.   This dependence on a dairy industry tends to grow as a country becomes more prosperous, because the sale of milk enables a farmer with very few cows to make a living.   Small farmers just cannot graze enough beef animals to maintain themselves and their families.

The other large source of food which can be arranged without the destruction of the animal arises from the production of eggs.   However there are prejudices in some parts of the world against the eating of eggs, and again the food used to feed egg-layers is of high quality and could be used more directly to maintain the food standards of human beings.

ANIMAL PRODUCTS USED IN INDUSTRIAL PROCESSES

Hides and skins

Leather is made from the hides of cattle or the skins of sheep, goats, and pigs. The value of hides and skins has fluctuated very greatly over the past twenty years, and there was a time when it was thought that leather could not compete with synthetic products. However, it has now achieved a scarcity value, and there seems little reason to doubt that it will command a premium price over the synthetic article so far as can be seen into the future. Naturally the quality of each hide depends to a considerable extent on whether it was damaged while it was growing on the animal or while it was being removed. There are many avoidable blemishes which reduce the value considerably. Perhaps the worst are holes along the back, and the most valuable part of the hide, made by warble fly grubs in the temperate climatic areas and by skin conditions like Senkobo disease or tick bites in the tropics. Carelessly placed brands can also ruin an otherwise good hide.

Hides and skins are preserved until they can reach the tanner in two different ways, and to a considerable extent the type of preservation selected depends on the weather conditions in the country of origin. In meat processing plants, and in wet weather conditions, they are preserved wet by placing a layer of salt over the connective tissue on the inside of the hide after removing as far as possible the small bits of tissue which remain there after flaying. They are then stacked one over the other.

The other way of preservation, and one sometimes used, is to dry the hides on a frame. They are stretched within a frame of poles by means of cords sewn through holes on the edges and left to dry in the shade. Those which are dried in the full heat of the sun, and on the ground, are much less valuable because they often wrinkle and dry unevenly so that stains appear in the leather after tanning.

Some skins are sold for the clothing and tourist trade in the natural state without being tanned into leather although they are softened by various processes. These are sheep skins complete with the wool and cattle skins with distinctive hair colours. This trade is very small and of little national importance. 'Persian lamb' skins are produced from newborn lambs of Karakul Sheep.

Wool and hair

There are two varieties of domesticated sheep, both containing many breeds. The most important are the wool sheep, and of these most of the wool comes from the fleece of the Merino breed. The hair or fat-tailed sheep are only used for meat, and then usually in those areas of the world where there is no organized meat industry. Mohair comes from a breed of goat, and other equally valuable industrial sources of hair come from the domesticated species of camels found in South America. Bristle is obtained from pigs but has been declining in importance in recent years. Wool fat or lanolin is obtained by extraction from wool before processing.

By-products of slaughter houses

Hooves and horns are made into glue; bones and blood are dried and made into bone and blood meal, both used either as food supplements for animals or as fertilizers. Certain hormonal glands are also detached and used for pharmaceutical purposes.

ANIMALS USED FOR WORK OR TRANSPORT

In many parts of the world, oxen not only supply the most economical means of transport on the farm but the one most frequently in use. They have the advantage that they can be fed off the grazing, but they need careful grazing management if they are to give of their best. Horses are still used outside areas where the greater part of the work has been taken over by tractors, and water buffaloes form a most useful and practical means of transport in areas in the tropics where the rainfall is high. The donkey is a hardy and useful work animal found in many parts of the world.   Other animals such as camels in the deserts, elephants in forests and sled-dogs in the polar regions have more specialized uses.

The principles of successful use of work animals remain the same whatever the species employed.   The quality of the food must be consistent with the amount of work required of the animal, and where this food has to be obtained from grazing then sufficient time must be allowed for the animal to feed and, in the case of a ruminant, to chew the cud.   Harness must be carefully examined to see that it does not chafe the skin, and the work asked should be of a type within the capacity of the animal.   Because working animals cannot seek it for themselves, water must also be supplied.   The sign of a good horseman is that he cares for the needs of his animal after a hard day before he cares for himself. This applies equally well to workers with other species of animals.

ANIMALS KEPT FOR LEISURE ACTIVITIES

One species stands out above all, in that it is almost exclusively kept for leisure purposes in the industrialized countries, and that is the horse.   Thoroughbreds are used in racing; other horses are used for show jumping, for trail riding or leisure riding.   Horses are held in high regard in most parts of the world.

The rise of popularity of spacious zoological parks is also a recent feature, and more and more are being developed in industrial countries with large city populations, and these contain both aquatic and land animal species.

The interest in game animals is reflected in the importance of game reserves and national parks, as a source of national income in the tropics and as confining areas in temperate countries.   This development raises some very special problems since many of the parks are situated in areas of human rural poverty, and tourist visits do little to raise the income of those who live near the parks, yet cannot use the land for agriculture.   There is little doubt that disease control and perhaps even treatment of individual animals within closely guarded parks will be of increasing importance in the future.

ANIMALS KEPT FOR SOCIAL PURPOSES

In all human communities as prosperity increases, so does the number of cats and dogs kept as pets.   There are very few exceptions to this rule, and it is therefore inevitable that pet animals will become a factor in more and more developing countries.   There is little doubt that the keeping of animals is socially beneficial to the human race.

ANIMALS KEPT FOR LABORATORY USE

There are arguments on both sides as to the propriety of keeping animals for experimentation and it is therefore very difficult to form an impartial yet sensible viewpoint.

Medicine remains more of an art than a science, in that while many factors in disease can be deduced on logical grounds, many imponderable problems arise in calculating the effects of a new treatment on individuals.   It is therefore commonsense to try out these problems on animals and to monitor the results.   Communities are hardly likely to refuse their sanction to the carrying out of animal experiments because past experience indicates that they are of value in saving human life.   However, the error arises in judging which experiments are essential and which are superfluous.   The humanity of those carrying out the experiments carries a constant responsibility.   They must not only judge the quantity of animals necessary to a result but its effects on the animals used.   They must constantly watch to see that there is no conscious suffering.

It is not too much to ask that each case should receive long and careful consideration as to whether the experiment is necessary and whether the stresses on the animals used can be reduced.   Undoubtedly, however, the public is going to be increasingly worried about this problem and the responsibility for seeing that the majority wish is carried out will fall more and more on the veterinary surgeon, supported by his technical assistants.

USES OF ANIMALS AND PRODUCTS OF ANIMAL ORIGIN

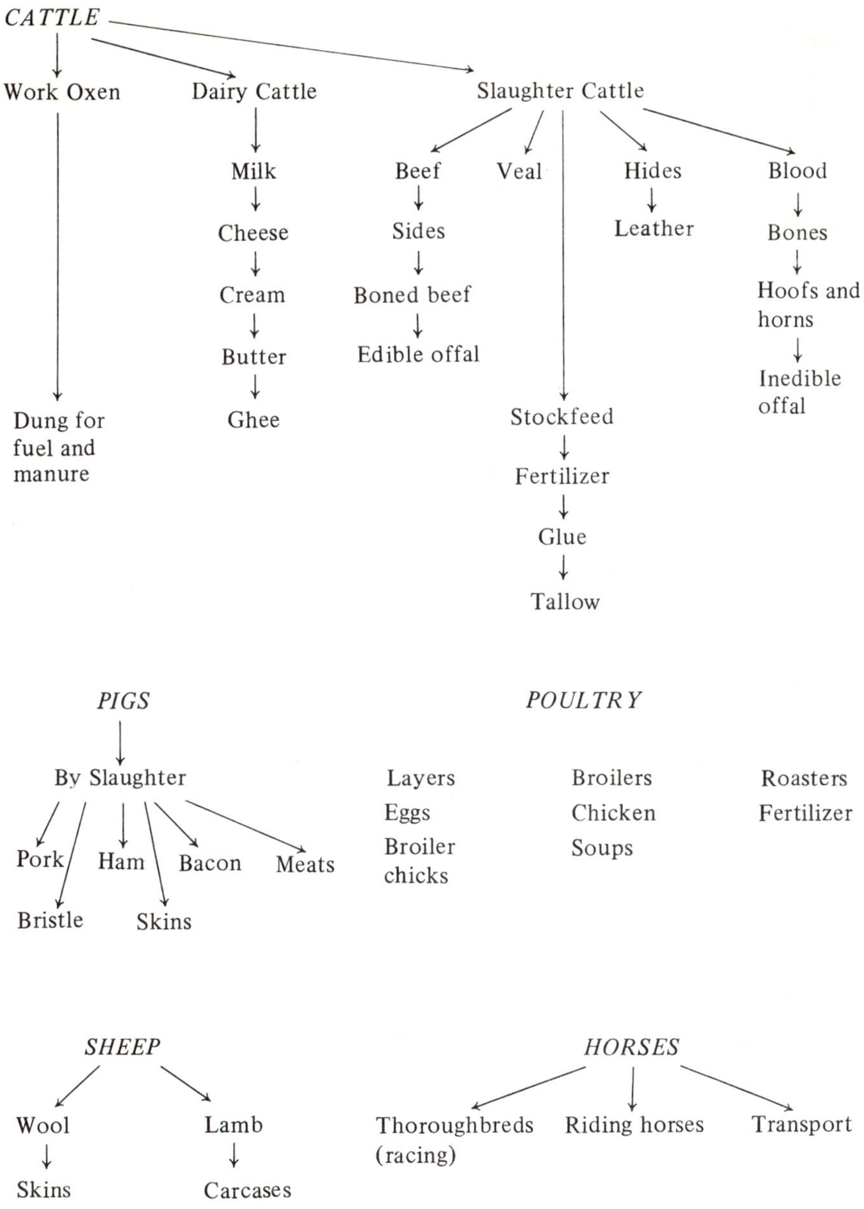

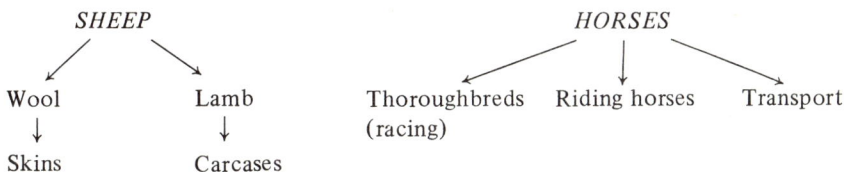

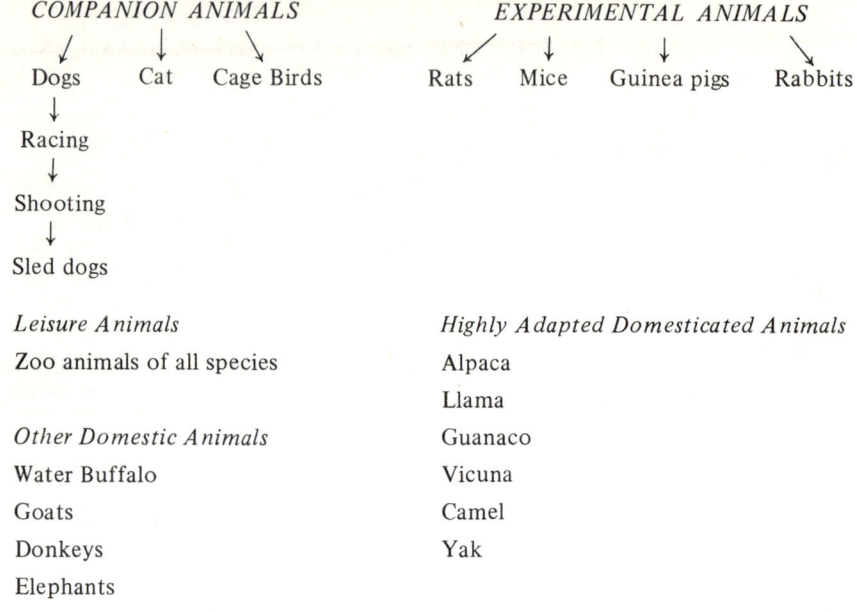

Leisure Animals

Zoo animals of all species

Other Domestic Animals

Water Buffalo

Goats

Donkeys

Elephants

Highly Adapted Domesticated Animals

Alpaca

Llama

Guanaco

Vicuna

Camel

Yak

SUMMARY OF THIS SECTION

(1) Man will continue to depend on animals into the future, and he is tending to be more dependant as time goes by.

(2) The requirement of animal protein for human food is increasing worldwide, and there is little sign that this need can be entirely met from synthetic sources.

(3) Sufficient food animals cannot be produced merely by feeding them on grass. To produce adequately, they must be given supplementary food.

(4) Beef is still the most desirable source of animal protein and is produced in greater quantity world wide than any other meat.

(5) To meet human demand for vast quantities of animal protein, a food animal needs to have the following characteristics—it must breed easily, cost little to feed, grow rapidly and be capable of living in crowded units.

(6) The other sources of animal protein are milk and eggs, but dairy cows and poultry must be carefully managed to produce economically.

(7) As communities become more affluent, they turn to animals to provide relaxation in their leisure periods.   Animals used for leisure or as pets are important to the quality of human life.

(8) All animals suffer from disease, and the control of disease is the quickest and most effective way of improving animal productivity.   It is the task of the veterinarian and his technical assistants to maintain the health of the animal population, no matter for what purpose it is kept, and the burden of this work is increasing and will increase into the future.

(9) Effective disease control is a combination of the maintainance of health in the individual, plus good management (provision of shelter, food and water) plus good selective breeding.

Section IV

The Relationship Between Health and Disease

INTRODUCTION

Quite apart from any humanitarian considerations it is in man's best
interest to keep his livestock in health and capable of producing to
their maximum capacity. In order that an animal may give of its
best, two separate factors are required. The circumstances must be
such that the animal is able to maintain itself in health, and it must
also be capable of taking in and utilizing the food that is given to it in
excess of that which it requires merely to exist.

Determination of health

It is extremely difficult to give a definition of health, but in practical
terms a healthy animal grows, reproduces, and behaves in a manner
which has come to be regarded as normal for its species and type.
Domestic food animals are asked to do more than merely survive,
they are expected to grow rapidly or to produce far more milk than
would be required by the young. Domesticated work animals are
expected to maintain a performance far in excess of any that would
be demanded by life in the natural environment. It is because man
demands so much from the animals under his care that disease is so
important. Blatant disease is usually easy to recognize; not only do
several animals in the same herd become sick but the signs such as
diarrhoea, distress in breathing, or pain are self-evident. This is not

to say that the cause is easily diagnosed, but here we are only discussing the departure from health. Even when only one animal is severely ill, we find little difficulty in recognizing the fact since we too can become sick, and we can identify with the animal.

It is, however, the chronic slight departure from health which makes the animal become what is usually known as a 'poor doer' that causes most concern. The only way to know when an animal is not behaving according to expectation is to measure its performance constantly. Careful recording of milk yield in cows will not only enable failures in health to be detected, but also physiological signs such as the imminence of oestrus or heat. Similarly, careful recording of the number of eggs produced by laying poultry enables the manager to see when disease is present, because either laying is delayed, or falls away from the level of production expected from similar birds at that time in the laying cycle.

The measurement of production

What therefore influences an animal in its growth cycle, and how may it be managed to give maximum production in its expected life span? All things have a beginning, a middle, and an end. The graphs of life spans of productive animals shown in the illustrations give the type of patterns that may be expected of our domestic animals. Some animals will do very much better than these patterns suggest, and some very much worse, but the graphs form a basis of comparison. In simple terms the essence of herd management is to breed from the best and to prevent the worst from reproducing themselves.

Given that these illustrations represent normal productive spans, what are the factors which influence those spans, and maintain the animal in health and full production? These influences can only be stated here in very simple terms but the measurement of function in animals is a very complex science, to which knowledge is constantly being added.

The requirements for existence in the natural state

Animals are very dependent on their *environment*. Because an animal maintains its temperature at $37.5°C \pm 0.6°C$ it follows that outside

THE ANIMAL AND ITS ENVIRONMENT

The Hazards

hunger—inadequate food—thirst—injury
poisons—neglect

Output: CO_2

Inputs: O_2
balanced diet of
carbohydrates
fats
proteins
minerals & vitamin
water

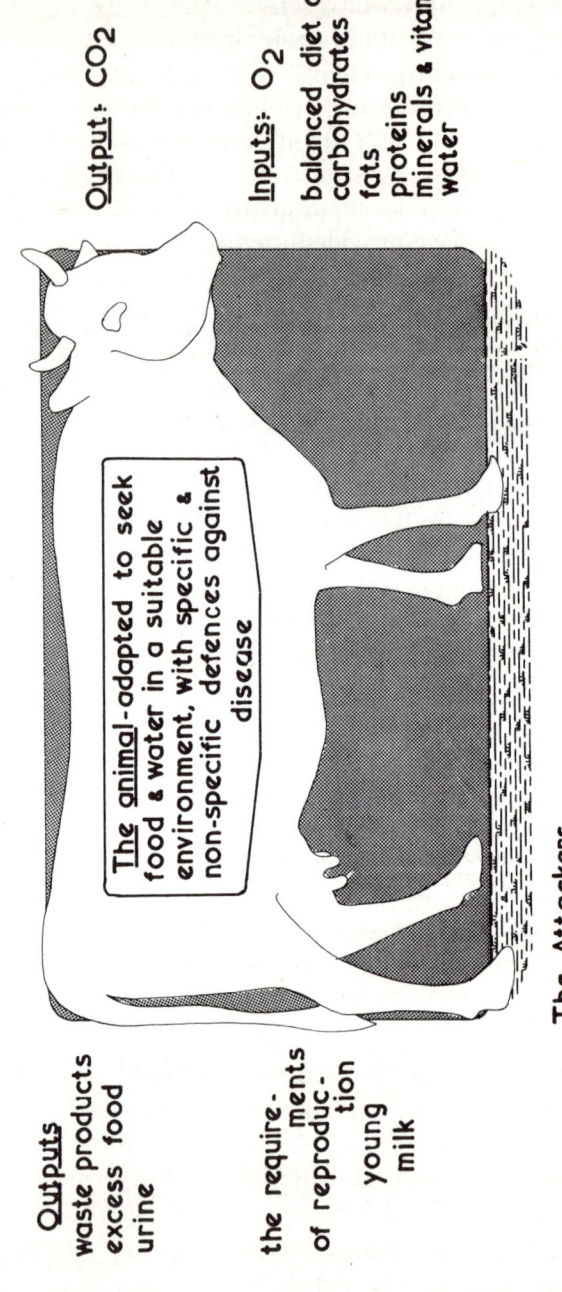

The animal-adapted to seek
food & water in a suitable
environment, with specific &
non-specific defences against
disease

Outputs

waste products
excess food
urine

the require-
       ments
of reproduc-
           tion
young
milk

The Attackers

viruses—mycoplasma—rickettsia—protozoa—bacteria
parasitic worms—insects—ticks—mites—predators

Figure 34

temperatures ought to be below that level for comfort; in cattle adapted to temperate climates a temperature of 25·0°C is probably to be preferred, and for animals adapted to the tropics one in the region of 30·0°C may prove more comfortable. Temperatures below this level will involve the expenditure of energy to keep warm, and those above involve the animal in water loss to reduce its temperature by evaporation. Naturally there are species of animals which have adapted themselves by the development of wool or hair to live in cold climates, and others which have provided themselves with greater ability to evaporate water and remain cool in hot climates. Most highly producing domestic animals have been developed in the temperate areas of the world, and their optimum temperature for growth and production tends to be well below blood heat.

Another aspect of environment is the presence or absence of wind, and the effect of the direct rays of the sun. Evaporation from the skin increases enormously in the wind, and hence the feeling of cold in winds of moderate temperature and the drying of the skin in hot winds. The provision of shelter from wind is therefore an essential in animal management. Similar effects are produced by the sun, its direct rays can product lethargy as well as photosensitivity in white animals. Shade is therefore another essential. Protection from rain is less of a necessity, more of a luxury; cattle tend to ignore rain which is not being driven by wind, provided that they do not have to lie on muddy ground in cold weather.

It is necessary at this stage, to mention the effects of stress. Stress is an unwarranted demand upon energy. It is quite impossible to remove all stress from the lives of animals but one can and should reduce it to the lowest practical level. To some extent the level of stress depends on the animal's normal behaviour, that is an animal which normally moves about in herds or flocks may be distressed if placed by itself. The most common causes of stress are, however, more self-evident. Failure to provide sufficient watering facilities is the most common, and transport under noisy conditions another. It is, for instance, a common observation that cattle are easily distressed by noise. In a slaughter house it is probable that it is the noise, and not the smell of blood, which causes the greatest disturbance and distress. A good manager is constantly wondering whether there is anything that he can do to reduce the wastage of energy through unnecessary stress on his animals.

A DAIRY COW'S LIFE

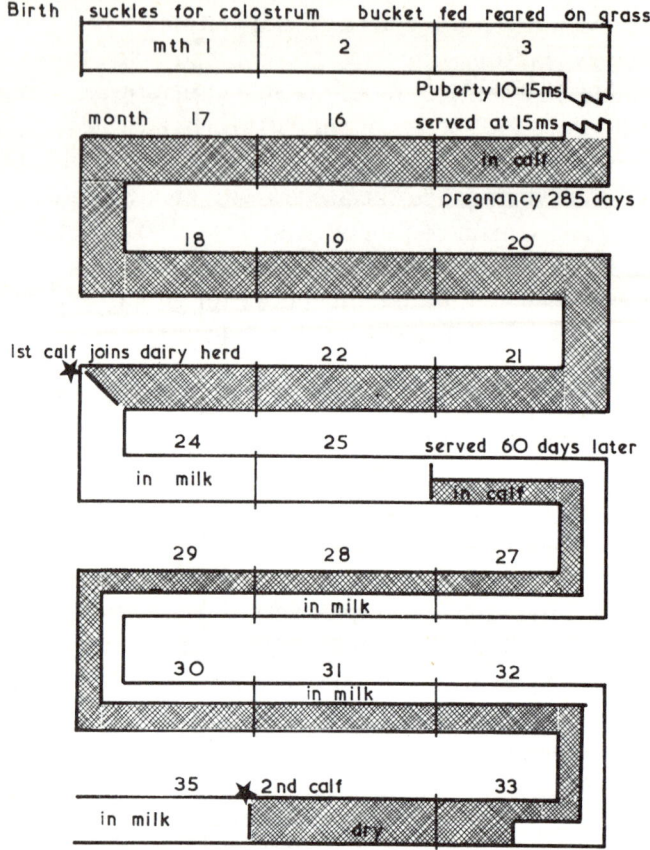

Average milk yield per dairy cow(U.K.) 905gals
Most cows are culled at 4·5 to 5yrs. of age
after 3 or 4 lactations.

Figure 35

The provision of adequate food and water

It is relatively easy to arrange to provide animals with sufficient water, or at the very least the most that can be provided in the circumstances, but the provision of adequate food is a different matter.   There

THE LIFE OF BEEF CATTLE

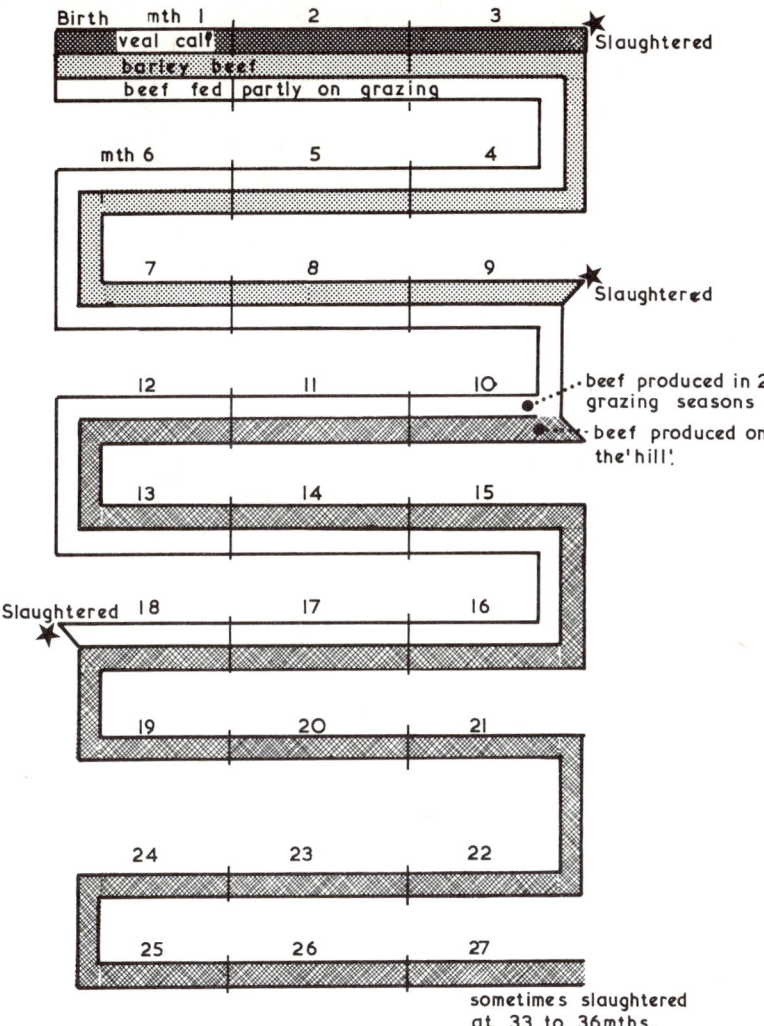

Figure 36

are three main constituents of all animal foods.   These are *carbohydrates* which are starches, sugars and fibre; *fats*, including oils and related compounds, and *protein* and other substances containing nitrogen.   The carbohydrates are mainly responsible for providing energy, the fats provide a reserve of fuel or energy within the body and the proteins are the body builders. The body works by means of a complexity of chemical reactions which draw their constituents from the air and from food and water, and such reactions require substances, often in minute amount to keep them in balance. These substances are either minerals or vitamins. A deficiency or in some cases an over-supply, of any one of these factors will produce at the least, a failure to grow, and at the most, frank disease.

Animals at work require more fuel than those at rest, and this fuel must be balanced between carbohydrates and fats to supply energy, and proteins to build up muscles. The same principles relate to the food producing animals, in that it is the balance of food components which are fed to them that determines the quantity and quality of the milk and meat that they produce. So far as grazing animals are concerned, the quality of the grazing is as relevant as its availability. Grazing is as good as farmers allow it to be. If pasture is over-grazed the grasses will be destroyed; if it is undergrazed, the coarser plants will take over and the grass will become tufted and less useful. Only so much production can be obtained from grass, partly because it grows in a seasonal cycle dependent on weather, and partly because it is difficult to maintain the sort of protein content in grass that is needed by the highly producing animal. To obtain the best potential production, supplemented foods must be supplied. However, such foods are expensive, and the decision as to whether to use them depends on the price that it is judged will be obtained for the animal when it or its milk is marketed. Judgement in this respect is assessed by agricultural economists.

The ability of an animal to respond to the demands made upon it

No animal is thought to have been domesticated for more than 8000 years, and at the time of domestication, captured animals were merely adapted to exist in their environment. Man has over the centuries improved on their natural qualities by selecting those characteristics which most suit his purpose. In addition he has greatly modified the characteristics which must have been found in the original populations. It has proved possible, or perhaps the urgency for selecting for changes has made it more essential, to develop some types of animal more than others. Furthermore this selection has largely taken place in the temperate climatic areas of the world.

There are many reasons for this.   Generally speaking, it was more difficult for man to survive in those parts of the world where the climate was subject to wide changes between summer and winter, and he has a greater incentive to conserve and improve his food supply. Another reason may well have been that by fortunate chance, wheat evolved in the fertile crescent of the ancient civilizations; that is in the biblical areas of the Middle East.   Once man had grain, he could concentrate on solving the problems of keeping sheep, goats and cattle.

The fact now remains that the breeds of cattle which produce most in the shortest time have all been developed in Europe.   This has happened over many thousands of years, and of course these animals give of their best in the climatic areas where they originated.   Outside these areas it is always a struggle to maintain them in full health and in production.   Zebu cattle (*Bos indicus*) are well adapted to the tropics but they have been subjected to far less pressure for change, and in consequence while they will survive in many adverse tropical environments they are seldom able to respond to intensive production methods.   In particular they are lighter in weight than European breeds of the same age, they are more seasonal in their breeding pattern, they give less milk, and their flesh, while more tasty, is less tender.   These are formidable drawbacks when the world is seeking more production from animals, and undoubtedly the future tendency will be for Zebu cattle to be kept in those areas where European breeds cannot be maintained economically. In short, the breeds originating from *Bos taurus* are likely to be found in more and more ecologically unsatisfactory surroundings, and the pressure for a strong constitution in these circumstances will increase.   The author's prediction is therefore that there will be increased selection of factors in European breeds which make them suitable for existence and production in the tropics.   Another factor will be an increasing emphasis on the control of tropical disease, so that exports of beef from the tropics and sub-tropics will become more acceptable to the other parts of the world.

The recognition of disease

It has been mentioned that blatant ill-health is not difficult to recognize, and it has also been pointed out that a low level of disease may only be determined by careful measurements of performance and by comparison with normal or average expected production.   However, there are many degrees of ill-health between these two extremes and there are recognized ways of detecting them.

The more one is familiar with an animal the easier it is to detect when it may be ill.   Normal behaviour in an individual is assessed by experience, and very often temperament changes may take place for no known reason.   Often these do not last for long, and may be safely

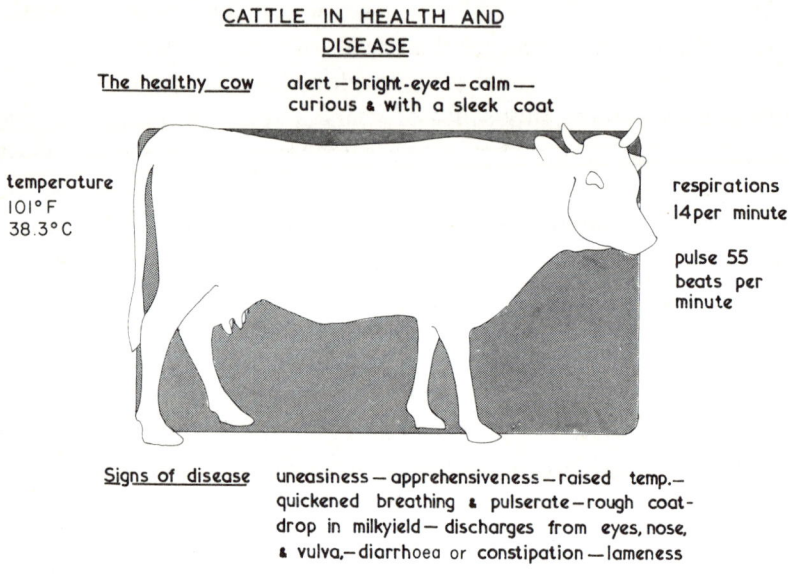

CATTLE IN HEALTH AND DISEASE

The healthy cow   alert — bright-eyed — calm — curious & with a sleek coat

temperature
101° F
38.3° C

respirations
14 per minute

pulse 55
beats per
minute

Signs of disease   uneasiness — apprehensiveness — raised temp.— quickened breathing & pulserate — rough coat — drop in milkyield — discharges from eyes, nose, & vulva,— diarrhoea or constipation — lameness

Figure 37

ignored.   The approach of oestrus in the female animal may produce behavioural changes, and must be discounted in an assessment of health.

It is not proposed in the following paragraphs to discuss injury in any detail, but it ought to be remembered that injury is the most prevalent cause of ill health in individuals.   A wound may be difficult to find if it is small and penetrating, and no one has seen it happen.

Recognition of a state of ill health

The recognition of ill health is of the greatest value if it takes place as early as possible in the disease condition.   The first pointer is a variation from normal behaviour, and commonly the first sign is a failure to eat.   There may be other factors which arouse suspicion, the animal may appear preoccupied, and stand or lie in a corner away from its fellows. The faeces may be looser than usual, and it may have an anxious look.

Detection of sick animals in an early stage of disease is only possible by patient observation of the herd.   Once cattle have become alarmed they rapidly lose any signs of apprehension and respond to the source of the disturbance.   It may be some time before they again return to their original uneasy state.

Once having detected an animal or animals in a herd by their abnormal behaviour one can proceed to the next stage.   Carefully separate the animals one wishes to inspect from the herd, and it is also good policy to include one animal which appears perfectly normal so that one can make comparisons.   It is quite impossible to assign precise rules in picking out such animals, because not only do signs vary between individuals, but a normal pattern of behaviour in one environment may be different from that in another.

The pattern of procedure

Most veterinarians have their own individual method of examination, but there are several ways in which departures from normal bodily function can be recognized.   Each one in itself means little since normal animals may also exhibit the same signs in some circumstances, but taken as a whole they build up a picture.

The most noticeable result of invasive disease is a rise in body temperature.   To be regarded as significant it must be at least two degrees higher than normal, in cattle this means over 39.4°C (103°F).   Details are given later of how to take a temperature.

A rise in temperature, whatever the nature of the organism causing it, produces in its wake several signs which, while indicative of disease, do not necessarily enable one to assign a cause.   These are firstly a rise in the rate of respiration, and secondly an increase in the pulse rate. Sometimes also there may be diarrhoea.   Watery faeces in the early stages of a disease do not necessarily denote an intestinal infection, they can be caused by general apprehension.

The first examination therefore merely detects that an invasive condition is present.   The next step is to decide whether it is an individual or a herd condition.   In other words whether it is infectious.   The fact that several animals are involved should give cause for concern; poisoning may affect several animals in a herd but there is seldom a rise in temperature.

The methods of diagnosis

This will be considered in two parts.   Firstly the methods that may be applied to the live animal, and secondly, those which may be applied at post-mortem.   At the outset it is emphasized that it is not always possible to assign a cause for every disease condition, and the depressing frequency with which the initials n.p.s. (no parasites seen) accompany post-mortem reports testifies to the difficulties of diagnosis.

Diagnosis therefore aims first of all to detect infectious, invasive, or destructive diseases.   In the absence of the determination of a specific cause it guides the process of prevention and treatment.   It also serves as a guide to *prognosis*; it is of the greatest economic and aesthetic consequence that the possibilities of survival should be carefully assessed.

The individual examination

The first step is to make sure that there is no injury, and no sign of swelling, and that there is no immediate potential cause of illness. Such things as the imminence of parturition, or the possibility of mastitis, or of obvious lameness should be taken into account.

If several animals are ill with high temperatures, whether or not salivation and lameness is present, seek professional advice without delay.

Taking an animal's temperature

Shake down the thermometer, moisten the bulb and introduce it gently through the anus into the rectum.   Using the weight of the finger ensure that it is resting against the intestinal wall.   Leave it in for half a minute, withdraw it and read the level of the mercury against the scale provided.

Taking an animal's pulse rate

In cattle this is commonly done by trapping the artery supplying the tail against one of the bony prominences of the coccygeal vertebrae

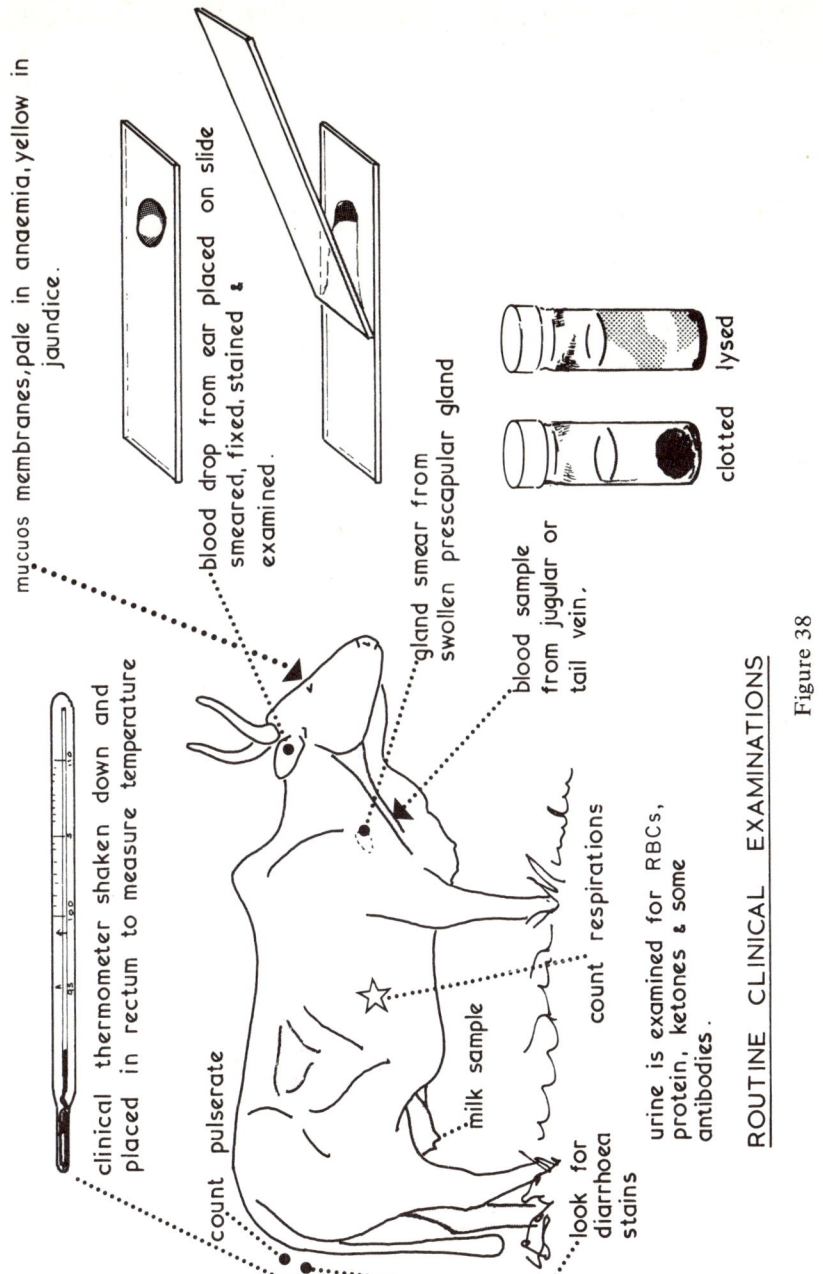

mucuos membranes, pale in anaemia, yellow in jaundice.

blood drop from ear placed on slide smeared, fixed, stained & examined.

gland smear from swollen prescapular gland

blood sample from jugular or tail vein.

clotted   lysed

clinical thermometer shaken down and placed in rectum to measure temperature

count pulserate

milk sample

count respirations

look for diarrhoea stains

urine is examined for RBCs, protein, ketones & some antibodies.

ROUTINE CLINICAL EXAMINATIONS

Figure 38

and counting the beats.   Most people count for half a minute and multiply the result by two.   Only gross increases are diagnostic in the resting animal.   The normal pulse rate in cattle is 55 beats per minute.

Observing the respirations and examining mucous membranes

The nature of the respiration is as important as its frequency.   Forced expiry or obvious distress in breathing cannot be missed but sometimes there are indications of difficulty that may indicate the first signs of pneumonia.

An examination of mucous membranes can be an indication of several types of disease.   Pale or anaemic membranes show a failure in the blood supply which may arise from true anaemia or from shock. Yellow membranes indicate the presence of jaundice and therefore a failure of the liver to function properly.

Examinations and specimens important in the diagnosis of tropical disease

The vast majority of animals in tropical and sub-tropical countries are kept under what would be regarded in temperate regions as extensive systems of management.   In short they are grazed, given little supplementary feeding, and are only housed for milking and protection from predators.

There is one big difference between disease conditions found in such areas and those found in temperate climates.   It is so important a factor that it can never be dismissed from any consideration of tropical disease.   It is the massive presence of arthropods.   The climate is such that there is rarely any relief for animals from attack by ticks, insects, mites, and sometimes leeches.   Sheer predominance of infestation by ticks or by mosquito attack can produce anaemia, but this is rare; the main cause of loss is the fact that many parasitic organisms from viruses to helminths, have adopted a life cycle which enables them to pass from one animal to another through the agency of an arthropod host.

Because these creatures do pass through a secondary host they are found in the blood stream since this is their means of reaching the insect or tick.   It follows therefore that they can be detected in the bloodstream by microscopic examination, and as a consequence no veterinarian or his assistant can function efficiently without a microscope.

The examination of blood

There are two ways in which blood can be examined.   The most commonly used is the examination of the blood plasma or serum for evidence of antibodies to specific disease.   It is however the other method with which we are concerned here.   It is the examination for parasites.

Diagnosis of disease by blood smear examination is not an easy procedure.   The presence of a parasite in one drop of the blood of an ox, at one specific period of time, either indicates a high level of infestation or a great deal of luck on the part of the investigator.   Nevertheless most infections produce a high level of parasitization and blood smear examination is a very necessary part of diagnosis.   The basic method is illustrated in the diagram, but it is a technique which improves by practice, and which is better learnt by demonstration. It is not proposed therefore to describe the process here, merely to point out that in the greater part of the tropics blood smears are an essential part of the veterinary art.

The examination of lymph gland and spleen smears

Neither of these techniques are possible in the live animal.   Gland puncture is frequently practiced in animals with noticeably swollen superficial glands but is usually a means of confirmation rather than the primary means of diagnosis.   Because these organs act as filters it is however particularly important to take fresh smears in the newly dead animal.

Post-mortem examinations

The diagram sets out the clinical tests which are routinely available for the examination of animals.   Apart from the simplest of these examinations, which largely involve clinical observation, most of them depend on an efficient back-up laboratory service if they are to be effectively applied.   The tests mentioned are applied to the live animal but there are routine examinations which are applied at post mortem, and if these are to be helpful, some idea of the reason for the collection of specimens should be understood.

Many post-mortem examinations do not result in an ascribed cause of death being determined.   Lesions detectable macroscopically (that is merely by observation) are the result of a long process of ill

health during life.   If the lesion is localized it may not show clinic-
ally in the animal's behaviour, but it will of course become apparent
on death.   It follows therefore that the more chronic diseases are
the most easily detectable at death, and that the longer the animal
has been ill the more easily will lesions be seen after death.   Remember however that an animal can suffer from a chronic disease yet die
of something quite different, and more acute in its effects.   An animal suffering from a chronic complaint is less able to survive sudden
stress.

MINIMAL POST MORTEM
EXAMINATION

SUDDEN DEATH   Eliminate anthrax and rabies.

PRELIMINARIES   Look for external injuries, emaciation, faecal, urine, and
blood staining.

THE EXAMINATION   Open down the mid-line, look at the abdomen first then
the thorax.   Note colour and quantity of any fluid present.   Note any
obvious changes such as swellings or distensions.

ROUTINE LABORATORY SPECIMENS   Preserve in 10% formalin in screw-
topped plastic jar.   4 mm thick slices of liver, lung, lymph gland, spleen,
through and across kidney.   Piece of stomach wall and/or intestine stuck
on blotting paper.

NOTE FOR LABORATORY   Name and address of owner, history of the case
and your opinion.

Figure 39

Very acute disease may therefore produce few obvious signs, but
by microscopic examination of sections from certain key organs the
process of investigation can be taken much further.   It is for this
reason that sections are sent to a laboratory for microscopic examination of the cellular structure, and certain tissues are common to
all such examinations.
The longer the animal has been dead the more decomposition the
tissues will have undergone, and to be of any value specimens for
microscopic examination should be taken from fresh tissues.   They
have to be preserved from further cellular damage by placing them in
a disinfectant solution.   The usual one chosen is 10% formol saline.
The container must be capable of travelling without spillage, it must

have a strong screw top, and is better made of plastic so that it will not break in transit. Sections of organ should be thin so that the preservative will penetrate them, not more than 4 mm in thickness.

The diagram explains the main tissues required but there are also organs needed for specialized examination—the general rules are as follows.

Liver—for detection of damage in the main organ of metabolism.
Kidney—for detection of damage in the excretory organs.
Spleen—for detection of blood parasites.
Whole heart or section including valves—should heart complaints be suspected.
Lungs—for detection of pulmonic conditions.
Abomasum or stomach wall—for evidence of inflammation.
Intestinal wall at the pylorus—for evidence of inflammation.

Bacterial examinations

Some of the most common diseases arise as a result of bacterial infection, and there are several routine methods used to type the organism.

Serological examination

As has been mentioned they may be detected by the presence of immune bodies in the blood serum or plasma. This involves the examination of body fluids, usually blood or milk, by testing their response to the specific toxic agent of the bacterium in solution. Most immune agents work by causing agglutination, or a sticking together, of protective agent and toxic component or antigen. This can be seen as a progressive cloudiness in the test-tube which can be compared with non-agglutinated controls, and with other concentrations of antigen. Several methods have been evolved of applying these tests on plates of agar in Petri dishes so that the degree of change can be more easily compared, and the test made more sensitive. Similarly field tests have been developed using drops of blood so that agglutination at certain dilutions is easily detected by a clotting of the blood cells.

Direct examination

Bacterial infections may be typed by direct examination, that is by staining matter obtained from a lesion once it has been spread on a glass slide.   The type of stain used and the appearance of the bacteria under the microscope being diagnostic of each type of infection.

Sometimes a sample (usually of milk) is incubated overnight so that the predominant bacteria proliferate.   It is then centrifuged and the bacterial smear obtained from the bottom of the tube is stained, and examined.

Biological examination

It is occasionally necessary to use laboratory animal injection in order to detect the cause of an infection.   Certain laboratory animals respond differently to infection with different types of bacteria.   Animal injection not only produces evidence of infection but determines the lines on which it should be treated.   The classic case is that of tuberculosis, when different strains of the bacteria can be detected by the differing levels of resistance exhibited to them by differing species of laboratory animals.

Resistance to antibiotics

For the sake of completeness the plating of bacteria on agar plates and the detection of their resistance to antibiotics is mentioned here. The object of all diagnosis is treatment or prevention, and the detection of the level of resistance of bacteria to different antibiotics is of paramount importance.   Unfortunately however the action of a bacterium outside the body is frequently different from its action within the body, but this is a different story.

The control of notifiable or designated disease

There are certain categories of diseases which can only be effectively controlled by a national policy.   The actual selection of those conditions which are thought better combated on a national basis varies between countries, but there are several diseases which are universally recognized as requiring international rules to prevent their spread.

Notifiable diseases fall into four categories:

(1) Those which by their presence imply a risk to human life. Rabies and tuberculosis are examples.

(2) Those diseases which are so highly infectious that productive animal management is extremely difficult in their presence.   Examples are foot and mouth disease and swine fever.

(3) Those diseases which disrupt the breeding pattern, and the fertility of the animals.   An example is brucellosis or contagious abortion of cattle.

(4) Diseases which lower the value of the products produced by the animal.   Examples are warble fly maggot infestation of cattle and Senkobo disease, also of cattle.

Reporting of notifiable disease

The detection of the presence of a disease likely to affect a country's economy or the health of its people involves an individual as well as a national responsibility.   It is of the utmost importance not only that the disease should be diagnosed, but that all the potential cases should be eliminated or protected by vaccination.

There is therefore a very present onus on animal workers to report anything suspicious of such infection to the veterinary authorities.

Disease in perspective

Most animals are healthy, and they stay healthy despite the constant hazards of their environment.   Even when they show signs of sickness these very signs may be the outward manifestations of a successful fight against disease.   The main object of treatment, and this will be said elsewhere in this book, is to provide the animal with the means of winning its own battle.   What it must have is water and succulent easily digested food conveniently placed near it so that it does not have to move far to drink and eat.

Disease when it occurs must be quickly recognized and promptly dealt with.   This is a matter for professional decisions, but the more carefully the technical assistant has recorded his or her observations the easier it will be for the veterinarian to restore the position.

ASSESSING THE HEALTH OF ANIMALS

Summary

The examination of animals should be undertaken in a progressive manner.

(1) Examine the behaviour of the animals from a distance. See which ones are standing apart from the herd and whether there are pain signals. Pain is shown in cattle by kicking at the abdomen, and by looking round at the flanks. General unease is indicated by cessation of rumination and standing away from the herd.

(2) A high temperature, combined with other signs, may indicate infection affecting the whole or part of the body.

(3) The commonly affected organs are those which interact with substances coming into the body. Breathing is affected by disease of the lungs, and constipation or more usually diarrhoea, follow upon disturbances of the intestine.

(4) Sick animals may therefore pant, or they may be stained below the anus from the effects of diarrhoea.

(5) Mucous membranes reflect the state of the circulating blood. They are pale or anaemic if the circulation of red blood cells is affected, they are coloured yellow if sufficient red blood cells have been destroyed to prevent the liver from removing the products of their disintegration.

(6) In countries and areas where blood parasites are common, a properly prepared blood slide can be a valuable means of diagnosis.

(7) Many animals will have a better chance of recovery if they are given individual treatment. In particular they must be given water ad lib and succulent easily digested food.

(8) It is wise to isolate sick animals from their fellows until the cause of their trouble can be diagnosed.

(9) Wash carefully, and disinfect clothing after contact with a sick animal.

THE COMPLEXITY OF DISEASE CONDITIONS AFFECTING ANIMALS

No attempt will be made in this book to describe disease conditions fully, but some appreciation should be gained of the complexity of the disease problem. Disease is by definition a departure from health. It may therefore be caused as much by neglect as by the effect of infective organisms. Good management is as important to animal production as are antibiotics and vaccines, and is as much a part of the effort to improve health.

The interplay of disease and health

Animals and man are in a constant state of struggle with their environment. For most of the time, and provided that there is sufficient water and digestible food provided, animals maintain themselves very well. However, during the course of life there are a number of periods when the animal body is less able to counter the trials that beset it.

Disease hazards at birth

The most important time is at the moment of birth. At this time the mother is particularly helpless; not only is she unable to defend herself from predators, but the mucous lining of the reproductive tract is open to the air and infection may result. In addition birth is a progressive series of events going on over a period of time. Firstly the fluids surrounding the fetus are expelled, this leaves the fetus in direct contact with the mother's reproductive tract, and its feet and head may damage the uterus or vagina. Next the young animal ought to be presented to the outside world head first so that it may have the opportunity of breathing as soon as possible after its connections with its mother have been severed. Malpresentations at *parturition* or birth are not uncommon and threaten both mother and the offspring. Finally the last act of birth is the discharge of the fetal membranes, and these are normally voided relatively quickly after the young have emerged. Delay in voiding the afterbirth can also be a hazard to the life of the mother.

The young animal is making the greatest change in its life. It is moving from a state where it relies entirely on its mother to one of independence. The first essential is for it to fill its lungs for the first time, and so stimulate the breathing reflexes. Next it must seek out the teats of the mammary glands to obtain nourishment. The first milk, which looks quite unlike the milk seen later, is very rich in substances which provide protection against bacteria and viruses. For a short time after birth the intestine of the young animal is adapted to absorb these complex proteins directly into the blood stream through the mucosal lining of intestine. This ability is rapidly lost, hence the absolute necessity for the *neonate* to have *colostrum*.

The disease hazards associated with ageing

Youth is a time when the animal is growing in body and in appreciation of its surroundings.   Its body needs food particularly rich in protein, as well as energy giving carbohydrates, it must also have the vitamins and essential minerals for its expanding body systems.   By contact with infective agents its body develops its protective mechanism against disease.   However this contact has to be kept within bounds, and too many hazards too quickly can rapidly prove fatal.   Similarly, curiosity can lead an animal into fatal encounters, and young animals are very curious.

Adult animals are usually well protected by previous experience against disease, but nevertheless they may be vulnerable to organisms which they have never encountered before, and infectious acute diseases are feared for that reason.   In addition it happens that a disease may become more invasive than usual, and by so doing overcome bodily defences that would be adequate to protect against the commoner low key infection.

Older animals become progressively less able to defend themselves in their environment, and hazards which would be of little consequence earlier in life assume far greater importance in old age.   Horses for instance are particularly vulnerable to leg injury, and, the older they get, the more difficult it becomes to heal the wounds and scars of hard work.

Diseases associated with crowding

Most disease conditions are harder to combat under conditions where animals are kept in close proximity with each other.   This is particularly so when young animals are kept in the same building as adults.   Diseases which may pass among adult animals almost unnoticed become quite catastrophic when younger animals are involved.   This is particularly true of pneumonias.

Disease conditions affecting both man and animals

Disease conditions which affect both man and his animals are known as *zoonoses*.   There are some very obvious and well known ones like rabies and tuberculosis, but many are less often mentioned.   Fortunately most diseases are species-specific in their effects, but there are many conditions which affect one species severely, and another only mildly. The big danger in such circumstances is that one species may act as a reservoir of infection for another. This is particularly important in certain forms of protozoal disease.

TYPES OF DISEASE COMMONLY ENCOUNTERED

Infectious disease

A disease is regarded as being infectious if it is caused by an organism which may be transferred from one animal to another. This classification covers the greater majority of classical or specific disease conditions. It might be helpful to examine in some detail the factors which determine whether an organism is likely to be *pathogenic*, that is a cause of disease.

Any one animal is a moving system of millions of cells adapted to its environment. It represents sanctuary to numerous single and sometimes multicellular independent organisms. Some of these parasites have become entirely adapted to life within another animal body, and have developed elaborate methods of reproducing themselves in such a way that their offspring may have the maximum opportunity of seeking a fresh host. Others are less specialized and may exist outside as well as inside the body. It may be considered that it is the more recently adapted parasites which cause disease, since to destroy the body may be to destroy the host, and their own means of existence. Whatever the philosophical explanation, the animal body is a system under constant attack from invaders. Some find a place within it and live in harmony, some are kept at a low level of invasion by the body's defences, and others may be completely repelled. The outward sign of that battle is provided by the state of disease.

The organisms which cause disease

Parasitic organisms cover the whole range from sub-microscopic particles of nuclear material such as viruses, to large creatures as ticks, insects and mites. They also vary considerably both in the length of time during their life cycle that they spend on the animal, and in their dependence on the host for their existence.

Viruses can only multiply inside cells and are found in the blood in vast numbers at the height of an infection, as they seek undamaged cells to invade. *Bacteria* have a more organized structure, and may either be entirely dependent on animal tissues to survive, or may be capable of separate existence in the soil. Some encapsulate themselves outside the body so that they may survive in a dormant state until they are ingested by a new host.

Mycoplasmas are branching structures which appear to be very primitive types of plants adapted to life in animal tissue. *Fungi* are a stage higher in plant organization but resort to the same method of spread in an animal tissue, while producing a specialized method of reproduction. *Protozoa* are unicellular animals which exist by invading and expanding within the mammal body. They frequently depend for the completion of their life cycle and the invasion of new hosts on the blood sucking habits of biting flies or ticks. Some have very elaborate life cycles in two hosts, the tick and the mammal.

There exists a whole variety of parasitic worms or *helminths*, some with simple and some with incredibly complex life cycles, which live in the bodies of domestic animals. The tapeworms or *cestodes*, for instance, depend for their continuing existence on their secondary stage—a bladder-like form—being ingested by a predator which has killed its host. The bladder develops in the intestine of the final host, and discharges its eggs into the intestinal contents.

Non-infectious diseases

Just as animals may be poisoned by an excess of a damaging substance so may they be harmed by the lack of a substance which they need in order to carry out their body processes. It has been shown that haemoglobin is probably the most important protein in the body, but this substance can only be formed in the presence of minute amounts of iron, copper and cobalt. Deficiencies of any of these minerals will produce a disease which shows itself in an inability to transport oxygen.

Dairy cows produce vast amounts of milk, and to do this they require large amounts of calcium and magnesium, as well as food constituents for use in manufacturing the factors which give milk its nutritive qualities.   High producing dairy cows may suffer from a deficiency of calcium and magnesium, and these deficiencies can build up to a life-threatening crisis very quickly.   Similarly it some- times happens that they cannot ingest sufficient carbohydrate to meet the demands that their udder imposes of them.   This again results in a crisis, and changes in their metabolism that produce disease.

Vitamins are complex organic compounds necessary to the correct balance of chemical interaction in the body.   The mammals cannot manufacture all of them in their own bodies, and are therefore reliant on plants to obtain their requirements.   A failure to get sufficient vitamins affects productive capacity.

The mechanical causes of disease

Despite all that has been said, probably the most frequent cause of disease is mechanical accident.   Machinery is becoming more com- plex and more widely used and inevitably there are accidents and animals suffer cuts, bruises, burns, scalds, and breakages of bones. As the number of chemicals in agricultural use become greater in variety and in application so do animals come more into contact with them.   Poisoning is a frequent occurrence, and probably more com- mon particularly at a sub-clinical level than is realized.

The concern about pollution is really a concern about poisoning.

PROTECTION AGAINST BACTERIAL AND VIRUS DISEASE: THE USE OF VACCINES OR BIOLOGICALS

The common invaders

There are two main sorts of living organism which enter the body and cause disease, these are bacteria and viruses.

Bacteria

Bacteria are small free-living cells organized rather like plant cells which harm their host animal by producing toxic substances.   Some of these toxins are attached to the body of the bacteria and cause

EXAMPLES OF DISEASES CAUSED BY ORGANISMS

Disease and species affected		Source of infection	Control measures
Swine fever— pigs	Virus	Highly infectious and contagious	Slaughter or vaccination
African swine fever— pigs	Virus	Highly infectious and contagious	Slaughter
African horse sickness	Virus	Transmitted by midges	Vaccine
Rift Valley fever— sheep and cattle	Rickettsia	Biting insects	Some vaccines available
Foot and mouth disease— all ruminants and pigs	Virus	Highly contagious and infectious	Vaccines only when slaughter impractical
Swine vesicular disease— pigs	Virus	Highly contagious and infectious	Slaughter or quarantine
Rinderpest	Virus	Most virulent disease known	Vaccines where slaughter impractical
Bovine malignant catarrh— cattle	Virus	Probably by insects	Slaughter
Transmissible gastroenteritis— pigs	Virus	Contagious	Vaccines of doubtful value
Bluetongue— sheep and cattle	Virus	Biting midges	Vaccination of doubtful value
Enzootic pneumonia— pigs	Virus	Infectious	Antibiotic treatment sometimes successful
Rabies— all animals	Virus	By saliva	Vaccination and slaughter of cases and contacts

Disease	Causative agent	Mode of spread	Control/treatment
Pseudorabies—pigs and dogs	Virus	Contact	Isolated cases difficult to control and impossible to treat
Scrapie—sheep	Virus	Chronic condition arising from contact	No treatment
Lumpy skin disease—cattle	Virus	Insects	Vaccine
Various poxes, species specific contagious ophthalmia—sheep	Virus	Contact	Low virulence
Heartwater—cattle and sheep	Rickettsia	Ticks: *Amblyomma* species	Broad spectrum antibiotics
Canine rickettsiosis—dogs	Rickettsia	Tick: *Rhipicephalus*	Broad spectrum antibiotics
Strangles—horses	Bacteria (*Streptococcus*)	Contact and ingestion	Antibiotics
Caseous lymphadenitis—sheep	Bacteria (*Corynebacterium*)	Contamination	Not attempted
Erysipelas—pigs, sheep and cattle	Bacteria (*Erosipelothrix*)	Contact and ingestion	Antibiotics
Anthrax—most animals	Bacteria	Contact and ingestion	Burn carcase, responds to penicillin
Clostridial infections	Bacteria	Contact—these are diseases caused by bacterial toxins	Vaccines
Bowel oedema—pigs	Bacteria (*E. coli*)	Combination of feeding and infection	Antibiotics
Salmonellosis infections—many animals	Bacteria	Infection by ingestion	Antibiotics, hygiene
Pasteurellosis (bacterial pneumonia)	Bacteria	Contact and ingestion	Antibiotics
Contagious abortion—cattle	Bacteria (*Brucella*)	Contact and ingestion	Vaccine, destruction of infected animals

Examples of Diseases caused by Organisms

Disease and species affected		Source of infection	Control measures
Tuberculosis	Bacteria	Ingestion and inhalation	Vaccines where slaughter impractical
Contagious bovine pleuropneumonia	mycoplasma	Contact and inhalation	Vaccines where slaughter impractical
Protozoal Diseases			
Anaplasmosis— cattle and sheep	Protozoa	Biting insects, ticks	Management and vaccination in controlled conditions
Redwater— cattle	Protozoa (*Babesia*)	Ticks, different species in temperate and tropical zones	Specific remedies insect control
Theileriasis (East Coast fever, Corridor disease, Mediterranean fever)—cattle	Protozoa	Ticks of varying species, life cycles of parasite often complex	Dipping, spraying
Trypanosomiasis (Nagana, Surra, Dourine, Chagas disease)— many species	Protozoa	Biting flies of various types but mainly *Glossina* species	Specific drugs or fly control
Coccidiosis— poultry, sheep, cattle and rabbits	Protozoa (species specific)	Contaminated ground causing ingestion of spores	Drugs and hygiene

harm when it dies and breaks up, and others are secreted by the bacteria and circulate round the body in the blood stream. The internal poisons are called *endotoxins*, and the external ones, *exotoxins*.

Viruses

Viruses harm the animal in quite a different way. They are composed of a protein found in the nucleus of animal and vegetable cells, called nucleoprotein. Viruses can only reproduce themselves if they enter a cell and induce it to produce more nucleoprotein, which is then taken up in producing more virus particles. The cell dies and the new particles are released into the blood stream where they seek out other cells to invade. As this process goes on very rapidly after infection, the course of a virus disease is usually swift; either the virus wins and the animal dies, or the animal wins and overcomes the virus. An added complication is that, because of the cell damage caused by the virus, bacteria are able to multiply with little hindrance from the body's defences by feeding on the dead tissue. Chronic ill-health following virus infection and due to secondary invasion by bacteria is therefore common.

Immune protection

The body's main defence against these organisms is to produce substances which can neutralize the toxins of the bacteria or destroy virus particles in the blood stream. These substances produced by the body in its defence are known as *antibodies*, while the substances which stimulate them into action and which are part of bacteria and viruses as well as other proteins are known as *antigens*.

It is important to recognize that each antibody is specific in its action against the antigen which has called it into existence. Any given antibody will only attack one antigen. There are other types of immune response but it is not proposed to discuss them here. Vaccines are produced to stimulate immunity to disease, and this may be *humoral* immunity arising from the presence of antibodies in the blood stream, or *cellular* immunity arising from an increasing capacity of specialized cells to absorb the offending organisms.

Bacterial vaccines

There are two types of bacterial vaccine. The first type is composed of either dead, or inactivated, bacteria; or, in some cases, of bacterial toxins so modified that they will stimulate antibodies but will not of themselves cause harm. The second type consists of bacteria which have been attenuated in some way so that they have lost their virulence and invasive powers. They will however still multiply in the body so stimulating antibodies which will combat them, as well as any more virulent organisms of the same type, which may later gain entrance into the animal body.

Dead vaccines are given in two doses. The first or sensitizing dose enables the body to start the process of producing specific antibodies, the second, or anomnestic dose, produces a far greater and more persistent antibody response. Similarly in an immune animal, the mechanism for protection is present although it may not be possible to demonstrate it by examining the blood, but nevertheless, the response to invasion by field organisms of a type against which it has protection, will be massive and overwhelming.

When live bacteria of attenuated strains are used to stimulate immunity only one dose is necessary since the organisms multiply in the body, and thereby produce the antibody response which eventually destroys them.

Virus vaccines

Virus vaccines work on exactly the same principles, and in a similar way; dead vaccines are better given in two doses, one to prepare the body to respond to the second and later dose. Live attenuated virus vaccine particles are given in one dose because they multiply in the body, so providing the stimulus for the specific antibodies that can combat them.

Commercially produced vaccines

High standards of production are required to produce non-contaminated effective vaccines which will not harm the animal, and many pharmaceutical companies produce commercial vaccines. Some are dead and some are live depending on the factors present in the organism against which it is proposed to produce a protection.

Virus diseases are frequently notorious, not only for having many types of casual organism, all of which have to be countered by a specific antibody, but also for changing their virus structure.   New strains of virus then appear, against which the existing vaccines are ineffective.

Allergy and anaphylaxis

The tissues of the body respond to all strange proteins gaining entry either through the skin, into the lungs, or by abrasion.   Sometimes there is an overreaction causing a rash, perhaps to an insect fluid, or perhaps shock from the injection of a strange protein against which the body has prepared defences but to which it over-reacts. Some people and some animals are more sensitive than others in their response.   The subject is a complex one, it is sufficient to mention here that allergy and anaphylaxis are both manifestations of the body's immune response.

Dogs frequently show the effects of an allergy after a bee sting.

EXAMPLES OF VACCINES AVAILABLE TO COMBAT DISEASES WHICH AFFECT ANIMALS

Disease	Details of vaccine	Domestic animals protected
Bacterial vaccines		
Anthrax	Live vaccine	Cattle, sheep and pigs
Salmonellosis	Live and dead vaccine	Cattle
Clostridial disease	Dead vaccines	Blackleg in cattle, and a wide spectrum of disease in sheep, mainly affecting the young animal
Brucella abortion	Live and dead vaccine	Cattle
Tuberculosis	Live vaccine	Cattle in areas where eradication by slaughter not immediately feasible
Leptospirosis	Dead vaccine	Cattle in parts of the world where it occurs—dogs
Virus vaccines		
Rabies	Live vaccine	All animals, but in varying strengths—dead vaccine is is also available
Distemper	Live vaccine	Dogs
Hepatitis	Live and dead vaccine	Dogs
Rinderpest	Live vaccine	Cattle
Lumpy skin disease	Live vaccine	Cattle
Bluetongue	Live vaccine	Cattle and sheep
Foot and mouth disease	Usually dead vaccine	Cattle
African horse sickness	Live vaccine	Equines

Section V

Methods Used in Treating Animals

INTRODUCTION

To the outsider looking in on veterinary practice the picture of treatment possibilities must appear extremely confused.   This is largely because he only gets a glimpse of the possibilities.   In the next few pages an attempt has been made to bring the subject into perspective, by painting in broad brush strokes the principles that underlie veterinary pharmacy.

Prevention versus treatment

The old cliché 'prevention is better than cure' is as true in veterinary medicine as in the sister science; however, to the old adage must be added the words 'and cheaper too', insofar as animals are concerned. Vaccines and toxoids are the sole agents available for the prevention of disease by active stimulation of the animal's inborn systems of defence against disease.

Sometimes antibiotics are falsely considered to be prophylactic agents, since it may be thought that continuous small doses over a long period of time will control infection.   To some extent this is true, and this method has in the past been used to stimulate production.   However, it is now universally acknowledged that the practice is bad.   It encourages bacterial resistance against the drugs used which extends in many cases to all other available antibiotics.   The practice leaves therefore few reserves of antibiotic for use if the disease happens to overcome the low levels used in its control.

The choice of a pharmaceutical

It is a sad fact that there are very few specific effective treatments. There are very many more than used to be the case, but nevertheless the conditions which respond to prompt treatment with a specific drug may be counted on the fingers of one hand. This leaves no excuse for not knowing which they are, and in each area it is important to know which disease conditions can be treated. Early diagnosis and treatment is always important in this regard as once tissue damage has proceeded to the point where repair has become impossible, no amount of effective specific drug will return the animal to normal.

Most treatment consists of a wise choice of medicaments which will combat the signs of the disease, the principal being that the animal must be given the opportunity of saving itself. Many of the old hearsay treatments, such as bleeding and purging, were not only ineffective but weakened the animal and prevented it from responding to the challenge of the disease.

It has been said many times in this book that diagnosis is the essential art of veterinary science. It is the choice of the right drug at the right time, or the decision to destroy, that distinguishes the good veterinarian.

The development of new products

While it is true that pharmaceutical companies are locked in a continuous struggle to produce new products, it is also true that this process is extremely expensive. It follows therefore that the major effort is directed towards the development of those products which have an assured market. There are few sectors of the veterinary market which are large enough in sales potential to warrant the major effort required not only to devise the products, but to test them and satisfy the rigid requirements of control legislation now appearing in many countries.

Most veterinary products are adaptations of products already successfully used in human medicine, the sole exceptions being the areas of vaccine production and anthelmintics. There is no point here in expanding on the troubles of the vaccine makers. In brief, however, it is sufficient to say that each batch of vaccine is an event unto itself, and a crisis can develop at each often-complex stage. Innovations can seldom be patented, and are easily copied, with consequent pressure on prices and interruption in the flow of new money to finance new innovations.

Successful pharmaceuticals are those which people will buy and, except in the dairy industry, there are few sectors of farm livestock production that will support the individual treatment of animals with modern effective but costly drugs.   There is therefore a restriction on the sectors of the market where real efforts are being made to produce new drugs.   It is an unfortunate fact at the present time that the treatment of tropical diseases of livestock is seldom worthy of protracted and intense research effort on the part of private industry.

Facing the facts about animal treatment

Knowledge of the course and causes of animal disease is constantly expanding.   In many cases it is emphasizing the importance of management in control.   However, in many parts of the world it is the application of known methods which is likely to be valuable rather than the seeking out of new methods.   Much of the knowledge is there; it is a case of applying it by using the methods now known and waiting for application.

TOPICAL APPLICATION

Topical preparations are intended to be used on the surfaces of the body.   This is a very blurred definition because for convenience all medicines that are not given by mouth or by injection tend to be included in the classification.

Dermatological preparations

These are substances which are intended for use on the skin, and a wide variety of drugs are manufactured for this purpose.

Farm animals suffer from a number of external parasites, that is fleas, lice, keds, ticks, and mites.   These parasites cause irritation but more importantly some of them transmit disease.   The classic example is provided by the tick.   In the temperate parts of the world ticks transmit virus and protozoal disease, but the climate does not favour excessive development, and ticks tend to be found only in very localized parts of the country, and so the diseases they transmit are seldom of national importance.   In Africa, however, not only are there many species of tick but they are seldom absent from any grazing area, and they transmit a variety of frequently fatal diseases. Perhaps the most important is known as *East Coast fever*.   It is caused by a small protozoan parasite which may be seen inside red blood cells or in the lymph glands of cattle during stages of the organism's life cycle.   It has been named *Theileria parva*, the first name deriving from that of Dr Theiler who first discovered its presence, and the second name meaning 'small'.

The control of tick borne diseases

The easiest way to control external parasites is to destroy them while they are on the animal, and many preparations containing substances poisonous to insects and ticks have been developed particularly for use in cattle and sheep.   Because of the need to treat large numbers of animals, and the importance of placing the poison in folds of the skin where the parasites are found, dipping tanks into which animals jump, and sprays which cover them with solution, have been developed.

Nearly all chemicals for use in dips and sprays are provided in concentrated solutions which have to be diluted before application. It is most important that the instructions should be very carefully read and understood before animals are brought into contact with them.   The interval at which they are used, that is whether the animals are to be treated once or twice a week or every second week, is determined by the life cycle of the parasite.   The important point is however, that *substances which are poisonous to insects and ticks are also poisonous to man and animals*, and they must always be treated with caution.

In general, dips are used for range cattle and sheep, while sprays are used for dairy cattle which might injure their udders in jumping into a diptank.   Animals must always be watered before entering a dip or spray race, and they must leave the area as soon as possible after most of the dip fluid has been drained away from the skin in the draining pen.

Other skin applications

Lotions and ointments mainly for use in dogs and cats are supplied in collapsible tubes, very rarely nowadays in jars.   They tend to be

TICKS—CONTROL BY BREAKING THE LIFE CYCLE

ALL adult females engorge
with blood and drop
to the ground to lay eggs

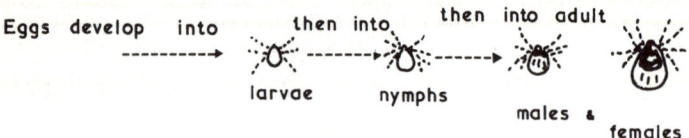

Eggs develop into   then into   then into adult

larvae   nymphs   males &
                                      females

Tick species are either:

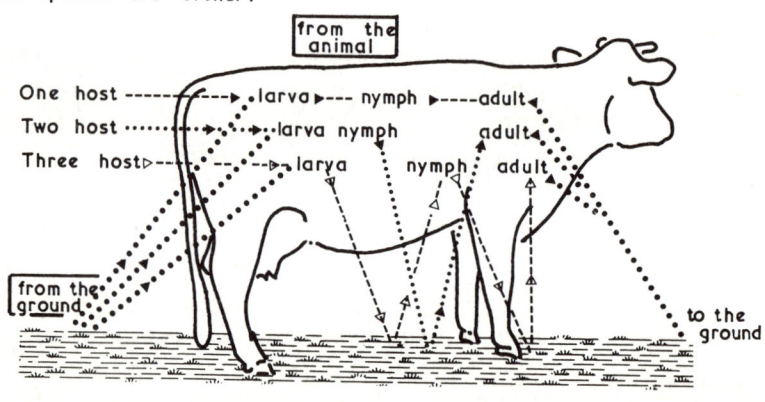

Ticks can only be attacked on the animal using dips & sprays

One host ticks spend more time on the animal than do two
and   three host ticks

Figure 40

expensive for use on farm animals where the main consideration is to prevent wounds from being pestered by flies.

Aerosols are frequently available; most of them contain antibiotic (see below, p. 152), and they have been largely developed for the treatment of footrot in sheep. They can be very useful for this purpose since they speed up the number of treatments that can be given in a flock. A simpler remedy may well be to provide a foot bath containing an antibacterial.

Udder preparations

The udder may be thought of as a very large skin gland which has been selectively enlarged in the milk cow by the breeding of animals capable of producing quantities of milk. The cow's udder has four quarters each served by one teat with one teat canal. Because it is so large, and because when it is full of milk it is so heavy, damage to the udder is very common. In order to counter this and the infection which follows a number of preparations have been developed which can be introduced up the teat canal into each quarter of the gland. They are known sometimes as intramammaries, and sometimes as cerates, but they are a means of introducing antibiotic, antibacterial, and occasionally anti-inflammatory agents into the gland to bring them into direct contact with the bacteria causing the disease. Intramammaries are used either during lactation to cure an acute infection or by introduction after the last milking to create a high level of antibacterial action during the dry period. The bases used for the two purposes are different. The acute cases are treated with bases which enable the antibiotic to be rapidly eliminated so that milk can be withheld from human consumption while the substance is present in the udder. The dry cow preparations are formulated in bases which allow for slow absorption from the udder into the blood stream so that antibacterial levels may be maintained for the longest possible time.

The selection of the right antibiotic to treat the type of mastitis, or udder inflammation, affecting the cow, and the best method to control the disease in a herd is a very complex matter. A great quantity of scientific effort and thought has gone into control measures, and it is often better that each herd problem should be studied by the veterinary surgeon attending the farm.

Mastitis is, however, a disease of production; low producing cows, or those which are merely kept in order to rear calves, seldom suffer from it.

Uterine preparations

It used to be the vogue to use a high proportion of uterine pessaries in cows, but present advice is only to use them in order to counter a specific infection, or on the instructions of a veterinary surgeon. Fertility, or the ability of a cow to produce a calf, is so important to its economic viability that nothing should be introduced either into the vagina or the uterus without the most careful assessment and in the cleanest of conditions.

Eye and ear preparations

Medicaments placed in the eye must be non-irritant, sterile, and must easily spread themselves along the conjunctiva. Most of the effective preparations are used in collapsible tubes with a narrow nozzle so that a small amount of the substance can be carefully placed into the cor-ner of the eye. Eye preparations should be placed nowhere else but in the corner of the eye, and then only when the animal is under restraint. There is otherwise a danger of damaging the cornea if the animal jerks away.

Ear (aural) preparations are usually made up for use in small anim-als; both dogs and cats are particularly troubled by aural irritation. Most of this trouble arises from seeds caught on the hairs inside the ear, but parasites may be present, and there is always a great deal of inflammation. The most commonly used preparations are probably those which contain a mixture of antibacterial, antifungal, antipara-sitic, and anti-inflammatory agents. As explained on previous occasions, however, a correct diagnosis is the shortest route to the quickest treatment. This is frequently a matter for close laboratory examination.

Surgical antiseptics

It seems appropriate here to mention surgical antiseptics, since in some ways they may be regarded as topical preparations. When an animal is subjected to an operation such as castration or ovariohyster-ectomy (spaying) which involves cutting into tissue, it is placed in danger of infection carried into the body on instruments or hands. For this reason all the instruments are sterilized of potentially harm-ful bacteria by several methods.

In a surgery this is done by prolonged boiling, or by superheated steam in an autoclave or by the use of chemicals which kill living organisms.   The easiest of these chemicals to use is alcohol, often in the form of methylated spirits.   The instruments can be stored in closed containers of alcohol until needed because it rapidly evaporates from the instruments when they are placed in air.   A variety of chem-icals are available to achieve the same end, but in general, while it is relatively easy to find a chemical to sterilize instruments, or objects, it is less easy to find one to sterilize the skin.   This is because a chem-ical in sufficient strength to do this often proves to be irritant and therefore does more harm than good.   It is a mistake to think that because a chemical produces a red flush on the skin it is being effec-tive; it may be irritant yet incapable of destroying the bacteria which are hiding in the minute skin folds.

SYSTEMIC APPLICATIONS OF DRUGS

The object of giving medicines systemically is to secure their circula-tion in the blood to the site of infection or to secure an immune res-ponse if they happen to be vaccines.

Medicines given by the mouth or in food are introduced into the digestive system; they may be absorbed in the same way as the food substances, or they may stay in the intestine and act on bacteria or worm parasites that are present there causing damage to the animal. Medicines which are introduced by injection either into veins, under the skin, or into muscle, are however being introduced into the blood stream and may therefore be expected to act very much faster than when given by mouth.   Naturally the fastest acting are those intro-duced into veins, and followed by those given intramuscularly, the greatest time lag between injection and effect occurs with drugs injected under the skin.

Medicines given by mouth or orally

Medicine may be given by the mouth in several ways, but in general it may be forced on the animal or it may be given in the food or the water.

Administration in food or drink

When medicine is given in the food, or as a food supplement, it must be acceptable. In other words, it must not have an objectionable smell, or taste bad, or have a different feel in the mouth from normal food. Animals are very sensitive to all these properties in their diet. If it is to be given in drinking water it must also be soluble. The main difficulty in giving medicine in the food is that if a number of animals are treated at once in this way, some will get more than others, because they are more aggressive in taking food or drink. It is impossible therefore, to give individual doses. So far as giving medicine to individuals is concerned, absorption may be poor when mixed with food, and one has of course to await the effect.

Administration by drenching

The other more individual but forceful method, of giving medicines by mouth, involves the use of pills or drenches. In the horse it is usual to give medicine using a stomach tube introduced through the nostril into the stomach. Medicine mixed in water is then poured into one end of the tube and will empty directly into the stomach.

Giving medicine using a bottle requires skill if the animal is not to be choked. The head should be raised and the medicine given a little at a time in the corner of the mouth by placing the bottle in the gap between the incisor and molar teeth. When the animal is seen to swallow, a little more is given, above all the animal must not be rushed, once it starts to take the medicine it will usually continue without trouble provided that patience is exercised. Some anthelmintics, or worm remedies, are given to sheep by a specially designed drenching gun which reaches into the oesophagus and gives the sheep a measured dose. Anthelmintics are also sometimes given to cattle by drench. When animals are sick it is better to give medicine by another method than by drenching, as the liquid is far more likely

to go down the trachea than the oesophagus.   This will cause coughing and, even if it does not damage the lungs, exhausts the animal to
little purpose.

Giving pills, capsules or liquid to dogs and cats

Oral medicines are far better given to dogs and cats in pill or capsule
form.   Many tablets nowadays are manufactured in a base which these
animals will readily eat, so that all that is necessary is to present the
pill to the animal in the palm of the hand.

However, the principle in giving pills to dogs is to hold the head of
the dog so that it cannot move.   The teeth are parted by gently pressing the gums at the side of the mouth against the back teeth using the
left hand which holds the upper jaw.   As the dog opens its mouth it
is held open by pressure of the second finger of the right hand on the
floor of the bottom jaw just behind the incisors.   The pill or capsule
is held between thumb and first finger, the head is held up and the
pill dropped onto the back of the tongue.   The mouth is closed and
the throat massaged, the dog should then swallow.   Cats can be
similarly treated but the claws of the front feet have to be watched.

Liquid medicine is given at the corner of the mouth with a spoon,
small amounts at a time being introduced at the commisures of the
lips, leaving time for the animal to swallow.

General comment

In the United Kingdom the prevention of disease by the addition of
antibiotics to the food is not allowed.   If animals are judged to need
treatment with antibiotics then this should preferably be given indi-
vidually, but, if this is impossible, then the dose used should be high
enough, and be administered for long enough, to effect a cure.   Sup-
plementation of food with antibiotics at a low dosage rate to act as a
growth stimulant is considered to be unjustified.

Medicines given by injection

Most medicines are now given to animals by injection, this is not only
because one can be sure that the medicine has been given and will be
absorbed.   Medicine given by mouth has first to be taken up from the

intestine, and some of it may be wasted since it may become mixed with other food substances and pass through the animal without absorption.   This is most likely to happen if the animal has severe diarrhoea or in the case of dogs if the animal vomits.

The methods of injection

Injections are made by means of syringes and needles.   The syringe is a tube containing a piston which forces the substance through its nozzle into the hollow needle attached to it.   The needle has a short point and is placed in the tissue into which it is desired to introduce the medicine.   There are different types and sizes of syringe, and the materials from which syringes are made vary according to the purpose for which they are intended.

Because syringes and needles are used to penetrate tissues it is important they they should not by accident, also take in infective bacteria.   Firstly, the solution containing the medicine must be sterile; this is one reason for using solutions made up in a factory because extreme precautions are taken to see that the injectable material is sterile.   Freedom from infection once the vial is opened is achieved by adding harmless preservatives to the solution.   Then the inside of the syringe and the needles must also be absolutely clean and uncontaminated.   Because of the great importance attached to these principles, many small animal injections are given using disposable syringes and needles.   These syringes are meant to be thrown away and they should *not* be stored and re-used.   It is practically impossible to sterilize them again once they have been used since this is done originally by irradiation.

Cattle syringes are usually of the multidose type and are made of heavy metal and glass.   This is to prevent breakages during use.   After use they must be dismantled and boiled for ten minutes or steam sterilized in an autoclave.   While it is not necessary to change the syringe after each injection, it is essential to change the needle regularly, and for intravenous injection one needle for each animal is a rule which should not be broken.

The routes of injection

The simplest type of injection is a *subcutaneous* one.   This is given under the skin in an area where it is loose and easily grasped in the hand.   In cattle the area over the ribs and just behind the point of the elbow is usually used.   A fold of skin is raised and the needle introduced through one layer of skin, the plunger of the syringe is pushed down and the solution thereby forced down the needle and left behind in the subcutaneous layer.   There is no need to rub the solution down nor to prepare the site by use of spirits on cotton wool.   Sometimes in nervous animals it may help to slap the animal in the area where the injection is to be given, or to use spirits to reduce the pain of the needle by dulling the skin.   Most cattle do not however react to the use of a needle of a sensible size.

PRACTICAL   ANATOMY   points of injection & treatment in the ox.

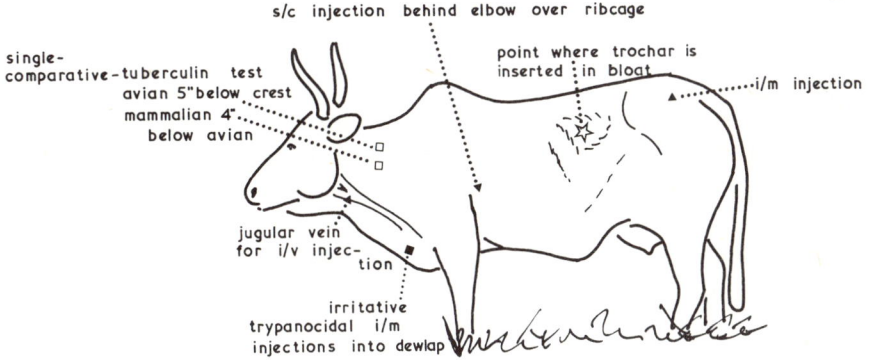

i/m - intramuscular
i/v - intravenous
s/c - subcutaneous

Figure 41

Intramuscular injections are given into muscles as the name suggests, but it is important that they should be given into the belly of a muscle and for this reason, in cattle the site chosen lies between the sacrum and the pelvis.   The main muscle in this area is known as the gluteus medius.   The action is to stab down with a 2·5 cm (1 in) needle through the skin and into the muscle tissue.   There should be no resistance to the injection of solution or suspension.   In the dog and cat, intramuscular injections are better given into the muscles lying in front of the hind leg rather than those lying behind the leg.   This is because it is very easy to inject between the muscles behind the leg and to damage the large nerves and blood vessels which run down the leg in this area.   Intramuscular injections require care if the solutions are to reach the correct sites.

Traditionally *intravenous* injections are given into either the jugular or milk veins in cattle.   However, and particularly in the U.K., the convenience of injection through the caudal vein has impressed itself on veterinary surgeons.   The site has many advantages over those originally chosen.

In dogs and cats the vein running close under the skin along the front of the fore leg is used.   No injection into a vein should be made without careful thought as to the effect it will produce.   The hazards are obvious of placing a substance directly into the blood stream which is going to be filtered out in all parts of the body through the capillary system.   Suspensions must not be injected by this route, because they contain particles which may cause obstructions in small blood vessels.   No substance which is suspected of being contaminated with bacteria should ever be injected intravenously.

Intraperitoneal injections are made through the abdominal wall into the peritoneal space, that is the space surrounded with peritoneum and lying between the abdominal organs.   This route is not used in cattle, and should only be used with great care in small animals.   In these animals practically the only substances so injected are anaesthetics, and present-day informed opinion does not entirely favour this route, preferring the intravenous method so that the dose can be more carefully judged.

The choice of injection route

Many vaccines are given by the subcutaneous route.   The only reason for not injecting a vaccine subcutaneously is when it is known to contain an adjuvant, that is a substance which will enhance its effect, but which might well cause inflammation.   The reason for choosing the intramuscular route in such cases is both to mask the inflammation, and also to place the material in a tissue well supplied with blood which will carry it gradually into the blood stream.   It often happens, however, that the inflammation shows up as a cold abscess at slaughter, this may particularly be the case when the dose is carelessly given. Anti-trypanosomiasis drugs are also introduced by this route and are notorious for producing this effect.   Intramuscular injection is used to give iron to very young piglets, and here again careless injection can produce unsightly healed cold abscesses in the muscle which reduce the value of hams at slaughter.

The use of the intravenous route, other than when inducing anaesthesia, is in order to give medicines which are needed in an emergency
situation in order to save life.   Examples are the use of hypo in
arsenic poisoning, and substances known as corticosteroids in cases
of shock in small animals.

MEDICINES GIVEN BY INHALATION

Relief from asthmatic conditions in man used to be sought by inhaling
substances which relaxed the tension in the small vessels known as
bronchioles which carry air to the lungs.   At one time small farmers
used to try this method on their cattle.   Fortunately cattle do not
suffer from human-type asthma but do suffer from pneumonia, that
is infection of the tissue of the lung at the point where air exchange
takes place, that is the alveolae.   Pneumonia is most commonly
found in calves around three months of age which have been moved
from one building or premises to another where they are to be
fattened for slaughter.   The combination of stress of the change, and
contact with infective agents to which they have no immunity, causes
disease.

Nowadays, there is no justification for giving anything by inhalation
other than an anaesthetic in a veterinary surgery.   The animal with an
infection of the lungs needs all the oxygen it can get, and it is quite
useless to expect any relief by using inhalants.

REGIONAL APPLICATION OF MEDICINES

Local anaesthetics are often used to block nerves which serve a foot
or the area of the rib or other very localized section of tissue.   Considerable skill is needed if they are to be applied with effect since to
be fully active the solution of anaesthetic must be placed around the
stem of the nerve, and a knowledge of anatomy is essential.

Poultices are a means of applying heat to local areas of the body;
they are made up from substances which lose heat slowly, and they
can be of great assistance in softening skin around an abscess to get
it to burst quickly.   The commonest poultices are made from kaolin
and glycerine mixed into a paste, but care has to be taken to see that
they are not applied too hot.   The test is whether the heat can be

borne on the elbow of the man applying them.   It is of course quite
useless to put them on animals which are not tied up.

THE PHARMACEUTICAL INDUSTRY

Pharmacology is the science of the action of drugs upon the body,
and a *pharmacy* is a place from which drugs are dispensed.   A *pharmaceutical* is strictly speaking a medicinal product developed as a result
of the science of pharmacology.   The industry has expanded greatly
in the last thirty years and has contributed enormously to the knowledge of medicine.   In this chapter it is proposed only to touch upon
the various pharmaceuticals that are readily available to the veterinary
surgeon today.   Vaccines or biologicals have already been mentioned.

TYPES OF MEDICINE AVAILABLE

Modern medicinal substances for animal use are as complex in their
production, and as potent in their effect, as those produced for
human beings.   Indeed many of them have been applied after prior
experience in human medicine.   The only truly veterinary products
are vaccines and anthelmintics.   Because they are so complex they
also tend to be costly, and their use on extensively grazed animals is
limited by economics.   Even where individual animals are concerned
the expense of treatment has to be considered and diagnosis should
be a preliminary to all applications.
    While simple remedies are less easy to come by, the value of nursing
on the chances of recovery remain as important an influence as ever.

ANTIBIOTICS

These are chemical substances produced by fungi which have the capacity in dilute solution to prevent bacteria growing or to destroy them.
Note that antibiotics are most effective against organisms which possess
a free life system, that is those which are complete cells with all the
properties of cells.   They are therefore of greatest value against bacteria, less effective against mycoplasmas and rickettsias, and have
little influence on pure viral infections.

Antibiotics are either narrow or broad in their spectrum of activity. Bacteria are divided for convenience of description into those which are Gram-positive, and those which are Gram-negative.   The Gram-positive bacteria are those which do not lose their colour when washed with alcohol after staining with Gram's stain.   The Gram-negative bacteria are those which are decolorized with alcohol after Gram's stain.   This change reflects a difference in the type of bacterial cell, and often in the type of disease which the bacteria cause.

Examples of Gram-positive bacteria are: *Bacillus anthracis*, the cause of anthrax, *Clostridium tetani*, the cause of tetanus, and all species of *Streptococcus* and *Staphylococcus*.   These last named are responsible for many purulent infections in man and animals.

Examples of Gram-negative bacteria are: *Brucella abortus*, the cause of contagious abortion, and *Salmonella* species, some of which cause diarrhoea in animals.

Narrow-spectrum antibiotics are those which attack either Gram-positive or Gram-negative bacteria; broad-spectrum antibiotics are those which attack both.

There is another important distinction in the way that antibiotics act; they either kill bacteria in which case they are called *bactericidal*, or they prevent them growing and reproducing in which case they are called *bacteriostatic*.   These two properties to some extent depend on dose, in that low doses are bacteriostatic and large doses bactericidal.   Note, however, that whatever the property of antibiotics outside the body, many behave differently within it.   This is because it is sometimes difficult to effect a concentration of antibiotic in the tissue or organ which is suffering from the disease.   Chronic bacterial lesions, perhaps caused by injury, are frequently sealed off by connective tissue and so protected from the antibiotic because the blood supply to such lesions is limited.   Sometimes also bacteria are protected because they are carried in the macrophages, or scavenger cells, which have engulfed them.   As has been explained tubercle bacilli are one such species.

Penicillin

The development of penicillin, the first modern antibiotic, is a matter of history.   It is extraordinary however that the properties which originally recommended it for widespread application still apply.   It is a narrow-spectrum antibiotic acting upon Gram-positive organisms, and it is particularly effective against rapidly dividing forms, it is therefore bactericidal in effect.   It is almost completely non-toxic and readily absorbed and can be given in massive doses.   Unfortunately certain people are allergic to it, and develop rashes when it is used upon them.   This effect would appear to have little importance or relevance in animals, except in the case of milking cows.   Here there could be a possibility of people sensitized to penicillin drinking the milk of treated animals.

Penicillin has been studied in great detail over the last thirty years and there have been a number of useful developments.   Notably the production of broad-spectrum semi-synthetic penicillins, which are effective against bacteria which have become resistant to natural penicillins by the production of penicillinases.   These are enzymes which destroy the penicillin molecule.

The first penicillin produced was benzyl penicillin.   This is very soluble in water and is therefore supplied in crystalline form in ampoules to which water for injection must be added.   Benzyl penicillin is rapidly excreted, and while high values are reached in the blood shortly after injection, these do not persist, and further doses have to be given.   This is inconvenient in use, particularly so in animals, and procaine penicillin was next developed; this is less soluble and is presented for use in a suspension.   Even this did not maintain blood values for a long enough period of time for convenient animal use, and benethamine and benzathine penicillins came into use which are even more insoluble, and therefore more slowly absorbed from an injection site.

The penicillin preparations for use in veterinary medicine are therefore:

Injections: Either crystalline for use after addition of water, or liquid suspensions which are shaken before use.

Intramammaries: Either presented in quick release bases for the treatment of cows in milk or slower release products for use in dry cows.

Ear and eye preparations: The non-toxic nature of penicillin makes it very suitable for eye preparations, but it has the disadvantage that it is ineffective against the rickettsias which cause one of the most intractable complaints in cattle.

Streptomycin

This is another of the early antibiotics.   It is narrow spectrum but this time acting against Gram-negative organisms.   It was originally developed for use against tuberculosis, and although bacteria rapidly develop resistance to streptomycin, it is still a most valuable drug.

It has one big drawback in that large doses are toxic, and may have a peculiar effect.   They may cause vertigo and deafness in man after injection, although these effects have not been described in animals. Its most useful application in veterinary medicine is by mouth to control intestinal bacteria.   It is not absorbed from the intestine, but attention has frequently been drawn to the bacterial resistance which develops in treated animals.

Streptomycin is commonly found in combination with penicillin in veterinary preparations.   This is because the two substances are said to be *synergistic* in action.   That is the combination of both products acting together is greater than each one on its own.

Streptomycin is available as an injection solution, frequently in combination with penicillin, and in oral preparations.   In this form it is particularly favoured for the treatment of bowel diseases because it is not absorbed from the intestine.   It follows therefore that when given in adequate dose by mouth the concentration of antibiotic in the intestine can be arranged so that it destroys harmful intestinal bacteria.   Neomycin, considered next, also shares this property.

Neomycin or framycetin

This is another narrow-spectrum antibiotic, effective against Gram-negative organisms, which possesses the useful property of being practically non-absorbed from the intestine.   It is frequently supplied as a mixture with other antibiotics, and sometimes sulphonilamides, to be given by mouth.   It can also be given by the intramuscular route of injection but it is apt to be painful.   It is considered by some to be too irritant to be used in intramammary preparations.

Chloramphenicol

This is the first antibiotic to be manufactured synthetically and it remains a most useful drug with highly valued activity particularly against *Salmonella* infections.   Unfortunately bacterial resistance builds up quickly when it is used in too low a dosage, and for this reason general advice has been to restrict its use to the most difficult cases.   It has valuable activity against rickettsias, and could be useful in treating heartwater.   It is better however to use tetracyclines for this purpose.

Tetracyclines

These substances have a very broad spectrum of activity ranging as they do over many species of Gram-positive and Gram-negative bacteria and over some rickettsias, mycoplasmas and large viruses.   The tetracyclines are bacteriostatic in action and resistance may develop if they are used in too low a dose.   Many of them were used in Europe in small doses in the food of pigs and poultry as a growth stimulant, the action appeared to be due to control of light subclinical or little noticed infections.

SULPHONAMIDES

These substances are regarded as antibacterials and have been in use in veterinary practice since the late 1930s.   In more recent years they have been superseded by antibiotics, largely because they are rather cumbersome to use and the ratio of effective dose to side effects is very low.   That is, relatively small increases of dose over that which produces the curative effects, are likely to produce harmful signs. The other big disadvantage is the rapid build-up of resistance by bacteria, so that they are not affected by dose levels of drug which would normally prevent them multiplying.   In most recent times a drug has been made available which is a combination of a sulphonamide and an antibacterial known as trimethoprim.   This combination has been found to be very effective against selected bacteria.

   There are many other antibiotics than those mentioned above, some are used for selected purposes and others are more generally used.   No doubt more will be produced, the important thing is however to understand that if they are not to be wasted they must be used correctly.   The principles are that:

(1) The right antibiotic should be used for the bacteria causing the disease.

(2) It should be used in correct dose.

(3) Dosage should continue in accordance with the manufacturers instructions.

(4) It should be used by the recommended route of administration. If in doubt read the packaging information.

CORTICOSTEROIDS

Introduction

The corticosteroids are hormones which are secreted from the cortex, or outer layer, of the adrenal glands, in response to another hormone which comes from the pituitary gland.

They were first discovered in the late 1930s and 1940s and their importance was realized by studying the symptoms of people who had suffered the loss of the cortex of the adrenal glands. These lie near the kidneys and because they excrete corticosteroids are of vital importance to the maintainence of life.

Since their original discovery, and when it became realized just how important they were in treating disease and shock, many substances more concentrated in their effect than those produced by the body have been synthesized. They represent a quite new departure in medicine, and their value in treating the individual animal is only just now being fully realized. They should never be used casually but in professional hands they can be life-savers.

The actions of corticosteroids

Corticosteroids have two main actions. The most important, but not the one used very frequently as a treatment in animals, is their function in regulating the electrolyte balance of the body fluids. It has been explained that all the fluids of the body are chemically buffered, that is, not only do they not become too acid or too alkaline, but any tendency one way or the other is rapidly corrected. Corticosteroids are the means by which this is arranged, by influencing the excretion of electrolytes.

Possibly the most valuable function is the control they exert over inflammation.   This appears to be achieved not only by constriction of peripheral blood vessels, but also by control over the production of white blood cells.   Medication for the control of inflammation has to be used with caution since the inflammatory reaction constitutes the first immediate defence of the body against bacterial invasion. In the absence of this response bacteria may not only multiply but gain access to the blood stream and cause a septicaemia.   Where bacterial infection is thought to be present corticosteroids should not be used without antibiotic cover.

Corticosteroids are widely used to control arthritic conditions in man and animals.

The topical uses of corticosteroids

It has been explained that corticosteroids reduce inflammation.   By this action they remove a sign of disease, not the cause.   Early in the use of corticosteroids in man their dramatic effect on the course of chronic skin lesions was observed.   Because of their value in controlling non-infectious human skin complaints, and because of the potential dangers of corticosteroids absorbed into the system, research was instituted into synthetic substances which would not be absorbed yet would still cure skin diseases.   Many of these preparations are now available for use in animals as well as in man.

In veterinary medicine they have their greatest application in small pet animals which are particularly prone to skin conditions in middle and old age.

Some final pointers on corticosteroid therapy

All corticosteroids should be prescribed with great care, it is for this reason that they are distributed only by veterinary surgeons.   In certain circumstances their use can delay healing, and in other circumstances they may interfere with the immune response of the animal to infection.   As a general rule the main danger arises during the course of chronic use, large doses can be used acutely without danger.

TREATMENTS AVAILABLE FOR PROTOZOAL DISEASE

Coccidiostats

The one protozoal disease found throughout the world is coccidiosis
of poultry. It also occurs in other species of animal but because
poultry are kept intensively, its effects among rearing birds can be
very devastating. It is probably impossible to keep poultry in economic numbers without using drugs to control this disease.

Coccidiosis affects the lining of the intestine causing it to break up
with characteristic diarrhoea and bleeding. The medicines used aim
at the prevention of multiplication of the organism, so they are known
as coccidiostats. If all the coccidia were to be destroyed, the bird
would acquire no immunity to the disease and treatment would have
to be continual throughout its life. As it is the coccidiostats are fed
in the early stages of the birds development and provided that it can
withstand the challenge from a heavily contaminated environment it
will acquire a good level of resistance.

One point to remember about coccidia and coccidiosis is that the
organisms are host-specific, that is each species of organism only
infects one species of host. The other point is that infected animals
rapidly acquire resistance and that the disease is only of importance
in intensive rearing conditions. There is one further point: the
coccidia also rapidly become resistant to the effects of any one
coccidiostat; it is important therefore to change the drug in use from
time to time.

Trypanocidal drugs

Trypanosomes are single-celled organisms which swim about in the
blood of the host animal. Most of them are transmitted by the bite
of a fly and some of them undergo a complex life cycle in the biting
fly before they become infective for the animal. The most widely
known disease caused by trypanosomes is 'sleeping sickness' of man
which is transmitted by the tsetse fly or *Glossina*. Cattle have been
excluded from wide areas in Africa by the presence of the tsetse fly,
but trypanosomal diseases of livestock occur outside Africa, in Asia,
and central and south America. Non-pathogenic trypanosomes can
be found in the blood of cattle in many parts of the world.

The difficulty with the treatment of cases of trypanosomiasis in cattle has been that while it is comparatively easy to eliminate the signs of disease with one dose of drug, given either intravenously or intramuscularly, the effects do not last and either reinfection occurs or the blood is not completely sterilized of the parasite. Research has therefore concentrated on the production of a longer-term effect, so that one injection will protect animals over as long a period of time as possible. The way this has been done is to give an injection of a drug which forms a depot in the tissues, from which the active ingredient is leached out slowly over a period of time. The difficulty has been to produce as inconspicuous and non-irritant a depot as possible at the site of injection.

All the trypanocidal drugs have been found to have some drawbacks. It is not proposed to discuss therapy here in detail, merely to show what drugs are available. As appears to be the case with all drugs used against protozoa, the development of resistance by the organism to the drug is a very great problem. It is often necessary to change the drug of choice in any particular area for this reason.

The suramin group of drugs were first used, particularly against Surra of camels, and proved very effective. Then the phenanthridinium group were introduced, the first being dimidium bromide, followed by ethidium bromide, and then by prothidium. The last one was used as a depot preparation for prevention of the disease.

Perhaps the most well recognized introduction was that of antrycide in the early 1950s. This drug is used in two forms, first as a curative in the methyl sulphate form, and secondly as a preventative by establishing a subcutaneous depot in the pro-salt form. Although some toxicity was reported, the drug still remains most useful.

Drugs which have stood the test of time are the diamides. In adequate dosage they will sterilize an animal of infection and also have useful effects against protozoa. They will do this even when resistance to other trypanocidal preparations has already become established.

Babesiocidal drugs

Babesiidae form a complex family of protozoal parasites which live and multiply inside red blood cells. They can be selectively stained in blood smears and show up as small blobs of coloured tissue inside the cell where they often take up characteristic forms which can be recognized. They are transmitted in the main by ticks, and many have a complex life cycle inside the tick as well as inside the animal body. Several species are of great importance in cattle as explained in the section on dermatological preparations, but one species is also of importance in the dog.

There are several well established remedies for the treatment of redwater (babesiosis of cattle) and babesial anaemia in dogs, but they should all be used in adequate dose and as early in infection as possible. Dogs in particular gradually acquire an enlarged spleen as a result of chronic infection, and this is a common cause of death in the tropics and sub-tropics.

Vaccines against protozoa

All vaccines at present available against protozoa depend on the infection of the animal with a small non-lethal dose of the causal organism. It is seldom possible to use a completely safe dose because of the individual variation in the ability of the animal to develop protective immunity. It is sometimes doubted whether there is any true immunity to protoza, protection depending on the animal harbouring a small number of parasites. There seems to be some mechanism by which the host can maintain a balance with the parasite and resist further and more lethal infection. This is known as a state of *premunition*.

TREATMENTS AVAILABLE FOR PARASITIC WORM INFECTION

All animals become infested with parasitic worms at one stage in their life time. The parasitic worm has an interest in seeing that it does not harm the host animal to the extent that it dies, so that left to themselves, most animals establish a balance whereby they do not disturb the few worms they harbour, and it would seem that the worms ensure that infestation does not increase to the point where the host is damaged.

However, this relationship is under constant test, in that, should the animal come under stress of very heavy infestation, it may suffer severely. Most worms have a life cycle which involves free-living

stages outside the animal body.   This is the means by which they continue their species in that they are constantly seeking new hosts.

Many of the worm life cycles follow the climatic seasons, and
attack the young animal at the point when it has been weaned, and is
beginning to eat adult food but has not as yet established its worm
balance.   It is at this time that worm remedies are commonly applied.
Since the young animal gains its worm burden from its dam, it is also
important.to see that adults are worm-free at the time they give
birth.

There are three common types of worm or helminths.   They are
known as roundworms or *nematodes*, flukes or *trematodes*, and tapeworms or *cestodes*.   Each type has a distinctive life history which
may be studied elsewhere, but there are certain points which are of
interest to this discussion.   All worm remedies are known as *anthelmintics.*

Roundworm treatment

Roundworms are the most common cause of disturbance of health in
young animals at pasture as well as in intensively fed stock.   The
simple remedies are cheap but highly toxic if given in too large a dose;
mixtures of arsenic were largely used at one time.   Nowadays, very
sophisticated remedies are available which attack the worms by affecting their ability to live in the intestinal tract.   Since most worms in
the early stages of their life cycle also move through tissues, the most
modern remedies will also affect these immature forms.   Modern
anthelmintics are not cheap to buy but, because they are effective,
enable larger and heavier animals to be produced from the same
quantity of food, and so pay for their purchase in increased profits.

Cheap drugs are frequently dangerous; effective modern drugs are
not cheap but safe and effective.

Treatment against flukes

Flukes are found in the liver and other organs of animals and are
difficult to dislodge without damaging the liver.   Part of their life-
cycle is spent in a snail, and in ranching terms, it is often better to
destroy snails by making sure that there are no damp areas in the
pasture than to try to treat the animals.   Remedies are available for

individual treatment, and this is more important in sheep than in cattle, but they are better given by injection. This is quick, less demanding of human labour, and effective.

Treatment of tapeworms

Tapeworms represent a paradox in that the animal which carries the final host, the recognizable tape of worm segments, suffers very little. Owners are frequently distressed by the presence of a tapeworm in their pets because it reproduces itself by shedding segments which appear in the faeces. These segments are full of eggs, quite large in size and have a squirming movement.

The true danger from tapeworms arises because they develop in the tissues of an animal which in the natural state would be eaten by the final host—the dog, cat or man. This secondary stage consists of small bladders found in many parts of the body of herbivores but usually in the liver or muscles. These bladders are sought for at meat inspection of food animals, and, if they are found, result in the condemnation of the carcase. Most bladder infection of cattle comes from infestation arising from human insanitary habits.

Remedies are available and effective against the tapeworms in the intestine of dogs and cats but no remedies are available to destroy the bladder stage in food animals.

ANAESTHETICS, IMMOBILIZING AGENTS AND ANALGESICS

General anaesthetics are those substances which cause an animal to lose its sensibility, while local anaesthetics are those which when applied to a small area cause a loss of feeling in the tissues served by nerves blocked by the injection.

General anaesthetics may be gaseous in which case they are given by inhalation or injectable in which case they are either injected intravenously (i/v) or intramuscularly (i/m) or intraperitoneally (i/p). The well known gaseous anaesthetics are chloroform, ether and halothane; the first is not now commonly used and the last (halothane) is better used in a closed-circuit apparatus. The injectable anaesthetics are either barbiturates (pentobarbitone, thiopentone, methohexitone) or steroids, (alphaxalone, alphadolone). The barbiturates vary in the time between injection and recovery and careful selection is necessary according to species and the type of operation to be performed.

In recent years a number of immobilizing agents have appeared on the market and these are most useful in controlling large animals. The one most commonly used through darts on large game is etorphine, which can be antagonized with diprenorphine. Xylazine is described as a sedative and analgesic for cattle; it has the advantage that the animal remains standing but oblivious to its surroundings. Another drug largely used in pigs is azaperone, also a tranquillizer.

Local anaesthetics are used to remove sensation when small operations are being performed which are potentially painful. Dehorning is one such example. They are injected onto the path of the nerves serving the tissue which is going to be cut.

In most countries operations on animals are prohibited without the use of an anaesthetic.

LIST OF PHARMACEUTICALS USED IN VETERINARY PRACTICE

Antibiotics: Presented as injectables, intramammaries, topicals (skin and eye, and ear), orals, feed supplements, inhalations, implantations, pessaries and suppositories.

Antibiotics available: Procaine, benzyl, benzathine and benethamine penicillin. Semi-synthetic penicillins—cloxacillin and ampicillin.

Streptomycin and dihydrostreptomycin. Chloramphenicol.

Tetracyclines—mainly oxytetracycline and tetracycline. Also chlortetracycline.

Other antibiotics available—neomycin/framycetin, tylosin, lincomycin, erythromycin.

Fungicides—griseofulvin, nystatin.

Sulphonamides: Mainly presented as oral products.

Chemotherapeutics: Presented in many forms according to pharmacological function.

Nitrofurans—tablets, powders and intramammaries for antibacterial and antiprotozoal use.

Anti-coccidials—amprolium, nitrofurazone, furaltadone, sulphaquinoxalone.

Babesiocidal agents—diamides, amicarbalide, dimetridazole, quin-
uronium.

Trypanocidal agents—phenanthridiniums, antrycide.

Anthelmintics: Mainly presented as drenches and feed additives,
but injectables are gaining ground.

Roundworm (nematodes) remedies—phenothiazine, piperazine
organophosphorus compounds, diethyl carbamazine, thibendazole,
tetramisole, methyridine, bepnenium, pyrantel tartrate.

Tapeworm (cestodes) remedies—niclosamide, benzanilide, arecoline
bunamidine.

Fluke (trematodes) remedies—rafoxanide, hexachlorethane, diam-
phenthide, oxyclozanide, nitroxinil, bromoxanide.

Ectoparasiticides: Usually presented as concentrations for dilution
in use in dips and sprays.

Simple—sodium arsenite, arsenic trioxide.

Anti-mange—benzyl benzoate.

Organic halogens—benzene hexachloride, diazinon, malathion and
other organic phosphorus compounds.

Neurologicals: General anaesthetics—inhalants (ether, halothane);
injectables (barbiturates, steroids, chloral hydrate).

Local anaesthetics—lignocaine, xylocaine.

Tranquillizers and sedatives—acetyl promazine and related compounds.

Immobilizing agents: Etorphine, xylazine, azaperone, diethyl-
thiambutene.

Fluid metabolites, foods and supplements: Remedial mineral
injections of calcium and magnesium, essential minerals—copper,
iron and cobalt.   Specialized foods and diets.   Vitamins.

Hormones and enzymes: Corticosteroids (ACTH, prednisolones,
beta and dexa methasones). Sex hormones (progestagens, oestrogens,
chorionic gonadotrophins).

Vaccines and toxoids: Live and dead bacterial vaccines and toxoids.
Live and dead viral vaccines. Sera and immuno-globulins

Disinfectants and antiseptics.

Anti-toxicants of various types.

Section VI

Emergency Treatment and Handling of Animals

FIRST AID

General considerations and introduction

First Aid is the help that is given in cases of accident to relieve suffering and if possible to return the injured animal to health. Specific disease causes dramatic losses among livestock but it should not be forgotten that accidents are probably responsible for as much damage and as many deaths. Accidents not only include damage to the individual but factors such as poisons which can kill a number of animals at the same time. It can sometimes be difficult to decide whether poison or disease is responsible for deaths and this too will be considered under this general heading.

There are very many ways in which accidents can cause damage, and it would not be possible to discuss all possibilities in detail here. There are however certain general principles which if carefully learnt will enable the reader to give immediate assistance when it is needed. It is hoped that the chapters on anatomy and physiology have been read and understood, since the successful use of first aid depends on a knowledge of how the body is made up and how it works.

One point must be made no matter how callous it seems. There is a big difference between human and animal first aid. The object of applying human first aid is to preserve life at all costs. The object in dealing with animals is to avoid suffering. It sometimes happens that it is kinder to destroy an animal humanely than to leave it to suffer from a long illness which might not in any case restore it to health and productivity.   Economic factors have to be considered and it may also be better from the owner's viewpoint that the animal should be salvaged as a carcase.   In which case the sooner it is destroyed and spared further suffering the better.   It is for this reason that this section contains a section on humane destruction.

Accidents—general principles

It is rare for a person skilled in first aid to be present when an accident first occurs.   Usually help is called and the helper arrives some time afterwards.   The most important factor when called to the scene of an accident is to remain calm; this may not be easy because those involved may well have seen what has happened, have taken sides, and be in a state of excitement.

Accidents to cattle and horses

First of all examine the animal carefully, note down the obvious wounds, but do not think that because an animal is off its feet that it is injury which is keeping it down.   It may well be in a state of shock, the effect of this usually being to make it indifferent to its surroundings.   It will probably have pale mucous membranes, and be breathing shallowly.   If it is lying down, first of all move it into a comfortable position, that is supported on the brisket with the legs in a natural, lying position so that it can breath freely and will not get blown.   This will enable an examination of the limbs for breakages.   Attempt to stop any arterial bleeding by applying pressure to the artery.   If the animal seems alright, apart from bruises and cuts, then leave it quietly to recover.   You may well find that it will rise to its feet in its own time and it can then be lead away to a place where it can be examined and treated properly.   Do not be confused by the presence of blood or even quite large flesh wounds; if there is no arterial bleeding and no bones broken then the chances of recovery are good.

Internal injuries

One must always be aware of the possibility of internal injury particularly where an animal has been hit by a car, and the opportunities for recovery must be carefully weighed up all the time.   It may well be more humane and of greater value to the owner if the animal were to be slaughtered and the carcase salvaged but do not be too hasty about this.   The main consideration in a heavy animal is whether a limb bone is broken, and where and how this has taken place; some fractures are worse than others.   Any persistent paleness of mucous membranes in the absence of visible bleeding two or three hours after the accident is not a good sign, and the animal must be carefully watched for signs of collapse.   If the animal is a cow heavy in calf then watch to see whether an abortion is likely.

There are other forms of accident than those caused by contact with machinery, and the most important of these is poisoning.   In many countries, animals are dipped, and great care must be taken to make sure that sick animals have not drunk the dip fluid.   In general, poisoned animals have all the signs of sickness, but do not have a raised body temperature which is the case if disease has caused the illness.   The most important first aid measure when poisons are suspected is to seek and remove the cause and to apply the relief measures explained in the section on poisons.

Accidents to dogs may be considered on the same general basis as above but the important difference is that a dog will readily survive a limb fracture, and can be removed to a veterinarian's surgery where it can be treated.

Cuts and bruises, burns and scalds

The thickness of the skin and amount of blood supply it contains varies according to the breed of animal.   This difference is most pronounced between *Bos indicus*, the Zebu breed of cattle, and the breeds originating in the temperate areas of the world known as *Bos taurus*.

Zebu cattle have developed in the tropics where in order to live they must be able to withstand the hot climate.   Their skin is very thick and is suspended in big flaps from parts of the body where it does not interfere with movement, below the neck as a 'dewlap', and in the region of the scrotum and penis in males.   This skin is well supplied with blood and the animal is kept cool by the constant radiation of heat from the skin that cools the blood which in turn cools the body during circulation.   The principle can be seen when a canvas water bottle is used, the outside is wet and the contents are kept cool by evaporation, whereas in even a dark glass bottle the contents gradually rise in temperature when it is exposed to strong sunlight.

Cuts in Zebu animals produce far more bleeding than is the case in other breeds of cattle, although it is probable that they heal more quickly. Cuts made by a metal blade may be clean and straight, but more often the objects that cause them leave a wound that is jagged and dirty. The most important thing is to clean the edges of the wound of dirt by gentle swabbing using a mixture of two teaspoonfuls of salt in a pint of water. Unless big flaps of skin are hanging down, the wound should not be stitched. Judgement must be made on whether the skin has a sufficiently good blood supply to keep it alive. Healing is known as 'first intention' healing when two surfaces of the cut skin are close together and tissue may be easily grown to join them. Healing of deep wounds comes from granulation which is explained in the section on inflammation and healing. Interference with the wound should therefore be the minimum to keep it clean; there should be no interference with clots and scabs no matter how unsightly they seem.

The exception to this principle is in deep dirty wounds when it may be necessary to give antibiotics in order to reduce infection from harmful organisms. Simple remedies will suffice for most wound treatments. Deep wounds involving muscle always look bad but as muscle is well supplied with blood healing is usually rapid and even when big holes in tissue are involved they will fill up more quickly than might be expected.

When arteries are cut the blood flows in bursts corresponding to the contractions of the heart. Small arteries can be stopped by the pressure of a temporary bandage but larger ones on the limbs may need the use of a 'tourniquet'. This is a piece of cord twisted round a limb and enclosing a pressure pad over the artery at a point nearer the heart than the wound. Tourniquets stop all blood supply to the area so they must not be left in place for more than half an hour. They can then be loosened slowly to see whether or not blood has clotted sufficiently to stop the flow; if bleeding returns, stop the flow by finger pressure and release the tourniquet for four or five minutes to restore circulation to other parts of the limb and then reapply the tourniquet for another period of half an hour. Most cut arteries occur in the region of the fetlock and the animal must be cast in order to arrest the bleeding. It may be necessary to apply surgical techniques in order to ligate the artery, but deep cut arteries in large animals are often difficult to find and ligate without casting and sometimes anaesthesia. It is surprising how quite large spurting arteries can be brought under control merely by applying pressure control from a roll of bandage tied in position.

Avoidance of flies

Another hazard to wounds is the presence of flies and it is necessary to use a good but simple fly repellent to keep them away. Stockholm tar is the old and still very good remedy but grease containing an insecticide is also very good and probably more easily obtained.

The comfort of the animal, and treatment of abscesses

Lastly the more comfortable an animal can be kept the quicker it will recover. If the harness is likely to interfere with the wound then the animal should not be worked. Food must be brought to it but most important it must be given as much water as it needs and it should if at all possible be put in the shade. Animals so left must be inspected regularly and the wound examined at least once a day. If there is any indication of its becoming infected then it must receive additional attention. An abscess may form and make its way to the surface or 'point'. The edges of an abscess are hot and painful, and pain increases up to the time when it bursts; this pain may be relieved by the use of a sharp knife at the *right time*. Wrap a piece of cotton wool around the blade so that it cannot penetrate too deeply then make a quick stab cut at the lowest point of the abscess. When the pus is released, open the wound only enough to allow any further pus which might form to drain, but do not close it or touch the layer of tissue which forms a lining to the abscess.

Treatment of bruises

Bruises are caused by damage which does not cut the skin but ruptures small blood vessels under it, causing it to darken in colour. Bathing with salt solution helps and then bruises will usually disappear within a few days. Abrasions are caused by rasping actions on the skin such as when an animal is drawn over a rough road in a car accident. Usually they look worse than they actually are, but the animal should be placed in the shade or kept warm as appropriate, and the road dirt

carefully removed by bathing with salt water.   In cases of extensive
damage, it may be necessary to inject drugs to prevent infection and
perhaps others to counter the shock.

Bite wounds are frequently surrounded by extensive bruising and
are often infected.   In such cases, it is necessary to use antibiotics in
order to counter the action of bacteria.   Remember the possibility
of the presence of a rabid dog in countries where the disease is
endemic.   It is rare for normal dogs to bite cattle, and, if there is any
likelihood of rabies, the report of a dog among cattle should always
be regarded with suspicion.   If rabies is confirmed then it is a worth-
while precaution to vaccinate the cattle with LEP vaccine as soon as
possible after they have been seen to be bitten.

Burns and scalds

A burn is caused by any object hot enough to kill tissue with which
it is brought into contact.   A scald is damage to tissue caused by very
hot water or steam.   There is no practical difference between the two
in their effects, and the treatment is the same.

The difficulty in healing comes from the fact that more tissue may
be affected than seems so at first inspection, or the amount of tissue
damage may be so great that healing will at best be slow.   There is
also danger of infection by bacteria which will grow in the dead tissue.
The first consideration in treatment is to remove the cause; thus if
the burn is caused by a sticky substance, this must be carefully washed
off with a salt-in-water mixture at the same temperature as the body.
Shock must be countered by keeping the animal warm or out of the
sun, according to the circumstances; give plenty of water and above
all keep it quiet.

There is great argument about whether burns should be covered
or left open.   To a large extent this depends on the circumstances,
and the comfort of the animal must be considered.   Bandages protect
the affected part from further damage but they do hide the condition
of the burn from inspection.   There is usually considerable seeping
of serum from the wounded surface and this as it dries provides a
protective covering, and when dirty bandages are removed this covering is also removed.   Bandages are not therefore bad things in themselves but in animals they are difficult to manage.   The principle
should be to interfere as little as possible with the healing mechanism

of the body.   Clean burns and scalds in the first place with a mixture of two teaspoonfuls of salt in water to get rid of dirt and damaging substances foreign to the body, then ensure that the animal is treated by a veterinarian to counter shock and to prevent infection.   The possibility of tetanus and its avoidance will be very much in mind in road accidents.

Damage to limbs

Cattle are heavy animals and they spend most of their life standing or moving to and from grazing and water.   The feet are constantly being bruised and damaged, sometimes this leads to conditions known as foul in the foot, but, more commonly, damage comes from nails or glass or through twisting as they walk among stones or concrete. The horn at the side of the hooves sometimes gets overgrown and has to be cut away so that the cow can walk normally.   Careful inspection will often show the cause of lameness and it can be removed and the foot treated.

Raising a foot

It is quite easy to lift and examine the front foot of a cow but the hind limb is more difficult.   If plenty of assistance is to be found put a piece of wood covered in sacking inside the hock and have two men one either side lift together.   If they stand close so that the animal feels itself supported then it will make little difficulty over the examination.

Fractures

Fractures are usually described as being:

Simple—a bone fracture with little displacement and damage to other tissues.

Compound—when other tissues are damaged and the skin over the bone is broken.

Complicated—when other tissues are damaged at the fracture site.

Depressed—when the skull is dented so that the brain or a sinus is damaged.

Comminuted—when the broken bone is in several fragments.

Greenstick—when the bone is bent rather than broken.

Impacted—when one fragment of bone is forced into another.

Multiple—when there are several fractures along the length of the bone or in other bones lying alongside.

The simple fact is that, no matter what the type of fracture, immediate problems arise of keeping large animals alive since they must move in order to eat. Dogs and cats are not only light in weight, and can be carried, but their food is concentrated and they can survive long periods of restricted movement.

Cattle have a large and complicated digestive system which must be filled with bulky food, and they are likely to blow if they have to lie down for long periods. It should also be remembered that cattle which have been down for periods of longer than a few days appear to reach a stage where they will make no effort to take weight on their limbs. As a general rule, particularly in the tropics, if the injury to a ruminating animal is such that it is unlikely to rise of its own accord within 48 hours then it is better that it be destroyed and the carcase salvaged.

Injuries to the jaw which prevent cattle from chewing the cud are almost impossible to treat successfully since the time to recovery is too great, and the animal will loose condition rapidly.

Bloat or blown in cattle and sheep

Bloat most usually occurs when cattle have been let out into fresh green pastures in spring or shortly after rain storms have occurred at the end of a dry season. The cattle like the taste of the grass and will gorge themselves; there is very little roughage in fresh growing grass, and it ferments actively in the rumen, blowing the animal out with the gas. Because of the complicated anatomical make-up of the entry of the oesophagus into the rumen, the cow cannot regurgitate gas under pressure easily. Typically the animal is very swollen on the left side, and tapping this swelling, which lies between the ribs and the point of the stifle joint, will produce a drum-like sound. Affected animals are obviously in pain and salivate profusely. Often a whole herd is affected. Animals left on their sides will bloat even if they have not over-eaten.

This fermentation is caused by living organisms acting on the grass, and the treatment depends on the type of symptoms that are seen. First, deal with the animals which are in greatest distress, one or two may well be lying on their sides. The need is to release the gas and this is done by stabbing through the skin muscle and rumen wall with an instrument known as a *trochar and cannula*; this is a metal tube enclosing a metal removable spike. The point to choose for stabbing is mid-way between the line of ribs and point of the hip some few centimetres down from the lateral points of the lumbar vertebrae. The trochar should be removed from the cannula when the rumen has been penetrated to the hilt, and, when the gas has escaped, the trochar is put back again in the cannula and the instrument is with-drawn. If no trochar and cannula is available, a knife may be used if the case is so bad that not to act is to leave the animal to die.

All the animals are then dosed with 30 g (1 oz) of 40% formalin or 120 g (4 oz) of 10% formalin in 0·5 litre (1 pt) of water. This is given in order to destroy the organisms that are causing the grass to ferment; 15 g (0·5 oz) of turpentine in 0·5 litre (1 pt) of linseed oil may also be used to gain the same effect. Sometimes the gas is in a frothy form and cannot be drawn off; the quickest way to relieve this is to give 15 g (0·5 oz) of any household detergent in water. The cattle should be walked around slowly until the gas starts to be dispersed.

Bloat can be easily avoided by only releasing cattle into new grass for short periods of time, and removing them from pastures which are causing trouble. The number of days in the year during which new grass causes a problem are very few in number and a little care in management at this time will prevent accidents.

Damage to udders and teats

The udder and teats of a dairy cow are frequently very pendulous and are subject to many injuries arising from scratches and tramplings, or to infections such as mastitis. Even quite small injuries to teats can cause loss in value to the owner out of all proportion to their size, because their presence makes the cow fractious and difficult to milk.

There are two specific conditions of teats which should be recog-nized; one is cow pox and the other is black spot. Cow pox is easily diagnosed since the sores take the form of little raised pits with an inflamed edge usually with a scab. Treatment of both consists of making the skin smooth before milking by the use of a softening cream, but there is no specific remedy.

Wounds on teats are treated with a milk salt solution or a cream which will prevent flies settling.

The most important type of injury to the udder is called mastitis, or inflammation. It has a number of causes but probably all start from an injury in the first place. If the cows are being hand milked it may be careless handling where the milker is trying to take every drop out of the udder and damaging the delicate membrane inside the teat canal as he does so. If the cow is being milked by a machine, then it must be properly set so that the strain on the teats is not so great as to cause injury. Most people with experience of mastitis think that the bacteria which cause it are present already, and that stress to the udder enables them to enter and infect the cells lining the udder.

Mastitis is probably the disease which most affects the productivity of dairy cows, and in consequence much expensive research has been aimed at preventing or curing it. This is no place to examine the problem in detail; suffice it to say that many veterinarians are of the opinion that frequently it starts in individual animals as a result of injury. It is noteworthy how rare the disease is in single cows kept by households for their own milk supply, and where the animal is regarded more as a pet than a milk machine.

Damage to eyes

The eye is one of the most sensitive parts of the body, and many animals are prone to eye damage. Cattle appear to be at greater risk than many other species, particularly at the times of the year when grass seeds are present in the grazing. There is also a specific disease caused by rickettsias which affects the eyes of cattle. It is probably transmitted by biting gnats in Europe and sweat bees or similar small insects in Africa.

A description of the eye has been given in the section on anatomy; however for the sake of completeness some facts are repeated here. The clear area in front of the eye is known as the cornea. It is covered by a thin protective membrane continuous with the mucous membrane at the edges, and known as the conjunctiva. The conjunctiva secretes a lubricating fluid which aids in the movement of the eyelids across the cornea.

In animals this is by no means the sole means of protection. In addition to the upper and lower eyelids there is a third, mucous membrane covered eyelid (known as the nictitating membrane) normally hidden at the inner corner of the eye. When the animal is healthy the eye is pushed forward from the eye socket by a pad of fat which lies behind it, but in sickness this fat is absorbed and the effect is to sink the eye in the socket.   This sinking allows the third eyelid to move across the surface of the cornea.   A similar effect is produced by gently pressing the eye back in the socket with the fingers.   The eye is also lubricated by tears entering the eyes from the tear ducts at the corners.   Tears have the same consistency as normal saline (0·9% of sodium chloride or salt).

Inflammation of the eye is accompanied by swelling of the tissues behind the conjunctiva, and by the injection of blood into surface vessels.   The eye becomes red and may be closed by swelling; white cells move across the mucous membrane onto the surface producing a milky liquid discharge.

These are all defence mechanisms aimed at removing the cause, but if they are unsuccessful, and damage to the cornea results, several additional signs are seen.   The cornea becomes cloudy, and an ulcer may form on its surface.   Because there are no blood vessels on the surface of the cornea, small vessels start to grow towards the inflammation from the mucous membrane, and of course sight is impaired. Damage may be increased by the animal rubbing against objects.

Inspection and first aid treatment to the eye

Conjunctivitis or inflammation of the cornea is commonly seen in cattle, and all the signs described are present, dependent on the extent of the damage.   Examine the eye by gently but firmly parting the eyelids using the first finger and thumb.   Pieces of grit or ulcers can be seen by looking along the cornea so that it reflects light.   Clean with warm salt solution, one teaspoonful of salt to 0·5 litre (1 pt) of water used in soaked cotton wool or with a fine hair brush.   If infection is present then one of a number of ophthalmic eye lotions should be used.   Cod liver oil and glycerine or olive oil can be carefully placed in the eye to cover the grit and enable the tears to wash it away.

The treatment of conditions of the ear

Inflammation of the internal ear, or otitis, is more likely to occur in small animals than in farm animals.   Dogs with flappy external ears, like spaniels, suffer because the ear canal is not exposed to the air and the discharge of sweat glands tends to be retained.   Other breeds and cats are frequently troubled by grass seeds, and the damage is compounded by rubbing of the source of irritation.

There is therefore no specific infective agent but a mixture of organisms all thriving on the inflammation which each one produces. The common start is an injury, perhaps from a grass seed; this causes damage to the internal ear surface and bacteria invade the damaged tissues. In addition there are species of ear mites which spend their lives in the ears of dogs and cats. The scientific name is *Otedectes cynotis*, and probably they cause little effect except in the presence of tissue damage. Because they feed on surface debris, clearly they are likely to increase in numbers if inflammation increases their food supply. By increasing in numbers they contribute to the inflammation. Fungi are also frequently demonstrable in damaged and inflamed ears, and again, while they have little impact on healthy tissue, they thrive in the hot wet conditions found in inflamed ears.

The most obvious first aid treatment is to treat the cause. This by no means as easy as it sounds, and it is better in the interests of the animal to seek the services of a veterinarian for the application of careful treatment, possibly under anaesthesia. The principle however is that all incipient signs of otitis should be treated as soon as they are seen to occur, and should not be neglected. The second most important point is to see that the ear is open to the air. *Under no circumstances poke about in an ear with a hard instrument.*

Snake bite

There are in all three types of snake venom; the type most commonly found will depend on the sort of snakes found in the area. The most dangerous are bites given by the cobra-like snakes which have hollow fangs in their jaws, with poison glands at the base of these teeth hidden under the gums. When the snake bites, it opens its jaw wide and the pressure of the bitten animal's skin on the gland automatically injects the poison. The poison from such snakes contains a neurotoxin which circulates in the blood and causes paralysis.

The effect of any snake bite depends on two factors—the virulence of the venom and the amount injected. Some snakes are more venomous than others. Cobra bites usually take place on the brisket front legs or head of the animal but the puncture wounds are difficult to find.   The only effective treatment is intravenous injection of snake venom, but the writer, after long years of experience, can recall no case where an animal has been seen to be bitten, has been so treated, and has recovered.   Cobra bite is usually diagnosed when animals are found dead and when no other cause of death can be found.

Another type of snake bite is that instigated by adders whose bites inject a venom which breaks down the red blood cells and cause considerable swelling of the tissues.   Adders, even the most venomous ones, are sluggish creatures, and in large animals the bites are usually in the front legs around the fetlock.   Dogs are commonly bitten in the head when they try to interfere with the snake.   Anti-venom should be used if available, but the use of corticosteroids in high dosage in dogs can often be dramatically successful.   Most dogs die of asphyxiation due to the swelling of tissues in the neck and difficulty in breathing.   Small swellings on limbs can be treated by bathing but the important thing is to treat the symptoms as they occur.   Infection usually follows at the site of the bite within a few days and antibiotics may be used to counter this.

The classic treatment of cobra wounds is to open the wound to the depth of the fangs, having applied a tourniquet to stop the local blood supply.   Clean out the wound, trying to get the maximum amount of bleeding below the tourniquet.   Most important, inject anti-venom immediately.   The tourniquet must be released after twenty minutes.

The third type of snake bite is that produced by pythons; these are simple non-venomous bites which crush rather than cut, and the bites can be treated as simple wounds.

Poisons

The study of poisons and their effects is called *toxicology*.   Many substances are poisonous when they are eaten in large amount or when they are given by an unusual route.   Some substances, which are by themselves harmless, may combine with others also harmless, to produce harmful results.   Toxicology is a very complicated subject and it is proposed here only to pick out certain common examples.

Arsenic poisoning

Arsenic has been known as a poison for many centuries and is produced as a by-product in the preparation of many metal ores. It was used as a dip for sheep in Europe for many years and is still the cheapest of the effective dips used to control ticks on cattle in Africa.

Nowadays arsenic is supplied to dips in drums containing 5 gallons of 20% soluble arsenic solution. This is diluted for use to give a 0·25–0·5% solution, the stronger solution being used in seven day dipping, and the lower solution in three or five day dipping.

It is probably true to say that all cases of arsenic poisoning in cattle are due to carelessness by human beings. Arsenic has a salty taste and cattle will lick it up when it is in its white crystalline form; equally if they are thirsty they will drink arsenical dip fluid. While it is possible to get arsenic poisoning by absorption through wounds in the skin, the main cause of death is by the mouth in food or drink. From this consideration arise some simple rules in regard to the safety of cattle at a dip site where arsenic is used.

(1) Cattle or sheep arriving at a dip tank should be rested and watered before they enter the tank.

(2) Fencing of the dip fluid store and the seepage pit must be kept in good order at all times. The cattle should only be allowed in the collecting pen, the dip, and the draining pen.

(3) Animals should leave the dip tank area to return to their grazing as soon as possible after dipping.

(4) They must not be rushed into the tank so that each animal may take its time in jumping. Care must be taken to see that animals do not push lighter ones under the surface, drinking dip as they go.

(5) Animals seen to drink dip must be treated without delay. *Never spray cattle with arsenic solutions.*

The treatment of arsenical poisoning

There are two types of arsenical poisoning, the first is called *acute*, that is the animal drinks a large quantity of the dip or licks up a large amount of arsenic at one time. The signs appear very rapidly, usually within a few hours and quickly get worse. The animal is obviously in pain, the stomach is tucked up, and it will get up and lie down again, sometimes groaning. At a rather later stage the diarrhoea starts, getting more liquid and blood stained. Treatment must be started as soon as possible.   There is a substance known as sodium thiosulphate (hypo for short) which when mixed with soluble arsenical compounds in the intestine forms them into insoluble ones which can be eliminated from the body with less damage to the tissues.   Soluble arsenic is rapidly absorbed from the intestine and causes great damage to the cells lining the bowel.   Clearly therefore, the sooner hypo can be given the better.   *Add 10 g of hypo to 100 ml of boiled filtered water and inject it intravenously into the neck vein, at the same time give a drench of 20 g of hypo in 300 ml of water.* These doses will only be effective if they are given within twelve hours of the time that the animal is seen to drink dip.

The second type is *chronic* arsenic poisoning and it is far more difficult to diagnose.   The animal will lose weight and may have diarrhoea, and it may be one of a number showing the same signs. There may be thirst and evidence of pain.   One way to tell these signs of poisoning from infection is by taking the body temperature which is lowered in poisoning, raised in infection.   If a number of animals are suffering from these signs, are known to be dipping in arsenic or are near a source of arsenic, and have a low body temperature then suspect poisoning.   Arsenic poisoning can only be positively diagnosed by examining body tissues in a laboratory.

Pieces of kidney and liver should be sent without preservative (10% formalin or other) to the laboratory.   The quantity of arsenic present in relation to the weight of the tissue will be assessed.   Animals regularly dipped will have absorbed small amounts, and this will be detected in the tissues, but levels higher than those regarded as average for the area will be symptomatic of arsenic poisoning. Note, however, that while in dipped cattle arsenic levels can always be found in the liver, this may not be the cause of death, and other possible causes must be eliminated.   Treatment is as described above together with the removal of the cause.

Lead poisoning

This is the commonest source of poisoning in cattle and has been reported from many countries and over a very long period time.   The main origin of the lead is from lead paints, particularly those used as primer paints on woodwork intended to be exposed to the weather. The signs start some three or four days after the animal has eaten the paint, this is because lead is slowly absorbed and distributed to the tissues.   The signs of lead poisoning are nervous in type and they may be confused with rabies in countries where rabies occurs.   They are usually described as bellowing in calves with staggering and frothing at the mouth.   The picture is also somewhat similar to that found in rabies and heartwater.   In tropical and sub-tropical countries it is therefore very necessary to deal with a possible lead poisoning case as one of rabies until proved wrong.

Plant poisoning

Poisoning from plants does occur, but the most important type has already been described.   That is *tympanitis* or blown, resulting from grazing on too fresh growing grass.   Certain other grasses, notably star grass, are dangerous when they wilt, because they release prussic acid at this stage, but poisoning by this cause is very infrequent. Plant poisoning is a rare condition and for that reason other possible reasons should be eliminated before it is reported as having been a cause of death.

Poisoning from the newer insecticides

The term *insecticide* should normally be reserved to describe substances which kill insects, and the word *ixodicide* used to describe substances which kill ticks, while the word *acaricide* is used to describe substances which kill mites.   Most insecticides are also effective as acaricides and ixodicides.   Because ticks, mites and insects tend to become resistant to these substances a constant search is made for more effective compounds, in particular for those with residual effect, that is substances which act long after the animal has been treated. Most of the substances which meet this need are organic compounds containing chlorine or phosphorus and they work by interfering with the nerve impulses of insects, ticks and mites.   An insect poisoned by one of these compounds becomes incoordinated in its movements, and eventually becomes immobile and dies.

It cannot be emphasized too often that in concentrated form insecticides can be very toxic to personnel as well as livestock.   Those handling the products ought to take extreme precautions to protect themselves and to see that substances are not spilt where animals have access to them.   The signs of poisoning in animals are nervous in type.   The animal becomes apprehensive, possibly because it does not feel in control of its muscles, it twitches and different groups of muscles may move in an odd fashion.   It also salivates, and there is an increase in the amount of tears formed.   Eventually the animal collapses in what is described as a fit, with incoordinated movement of the legs, neck and tail.   Treatment, to be effective, must be given early, recovery from severe cases is uncommon.

Commonly available organic compounds used as dips and sprays are DDT, BHC or Gammotox, Toxaphene and Delnav.   All are effective compounds used in the correct concentration but it must be remembered that they are effective because they are poisonous.   The antidotes are substances known as oximes, PAM for short, used in conjunction with atropine.

Strychnine poisoning

Strychnine is a very effective poison for the destruction of vermin such as foxes, jackals, and hyaenas.   It has been used to try to reduce wild carnivorous animals in areas where rabies is present.   Usually it is given in meat, but if this is done the most rigid precautions must be taken to see that people and dogs and cats do not eat the bait. Each piece of meat treated with strychnine should be marked, and each bait should be examined at regular intervals to see whether it has been eaten.   The bait should be laid after careful consideration of the habits of the animal which it is desired to destroy; there is little justification for putting out such baits in daytime.   They should therefore be laid out at nightfall and taken in at dawn.   An attempt should be made to trace any animal which has eaten a bait.

The symptoms of strychnine poisoning are extreme rigidity of muscles with spasms of acute contraction of all voluntary muscles. There is defaecation and urination, and death takes place very rapidly.   It is quite useless to apply antidotes.   Strychnine is very bitter in taste, and is usually only eaten by animals which bolt their food such as dogs, jackals, hyaenas and scavenging birds like vultures.

Salt poisoning

Salt poisoning used to be quite common in pigs due to people giving salty food while restricting the amount of water available to the animals.   *Salt poisoning is impossible if plentiful amounts of fresh water are available.*   Pigs which have received too much salt have the electrolyte balance of their blood and tissue fluids altered, and water is drawn into the intestines. This results in watery diarrhoea, excessive salivation, and staggering.

The remedy is to supply as much clean drinking water as the animal will take. Sometimes salt poisoning is difficult to diagnose because the source may be outside the owner's control and may have leaked into the water supply. Poultry may also suffer from salt poisoning.

Effect of rat poison on dogs and cats

Rat poison will cause death in dogs and cats and when these poisons are being used in buildings care should be taken to keep pets out until all the poison baits have been either taken by rats or removed. Various types of poison are used. The phosphorus type, e.g. Rodine, causes damage to dog and cat livers; the animals vomit and have inflammation of the bowel, becoming jaundiced as a result of liver damage. The warfarin type causes haemorrhages in all animal tissues and post-mortem examination shows areas of unclotted blood in the tissues. The red squill type causes vomiting and paralysis.

Rat poisons are sometimes used maliciously by people who wish to get rid of a dog, but one should always be very careful not to say that a dog has been poisoned until the laboratory has confirmed the presence of poison in the stomach contents.

Poisoning from nitrates used as fertilizers

Fertilizers are added to the soil to provide nitrogen for growing plants. Normally they pass into the soil and are taken up by the plants to improve crop yield and grazing; however, sometimes they are spilled and since some forms have the appearance of salt they may be eaten by animals. Very occasionally they may be mixed into animal food by people who think that they are adding salt.

Nitrates act in two ways in the body. They may be absorbed and passed through the kidneys, causing severe damage, with inflammation of the kidney structure, and interfering with the excretion of waste products. Sometimes they are absorbed as nitrites from the intestine and affect the blood, preventing the transport of oxygen. There is no treatment and diagnosis is often difficult unless the source of nitrite can be found.   The best form of prevention is to make sure that fertilizers are never kept in the same building as animal food.

THE RESTRAINT AND NURSING OF ANIMALS

In the thousands of years since man first domesticated animals, he has selected for breeding those individuals which are most likely to conform to his requirements, if possible without aggression.   Nevertheless, large domesticated animals have to be handled with respect for their size, and this applies particularly when they are sick.   Many hunters have recorded that wild animals which are sick from a disease such as rinderpest will charge without provocation.   It may be that such animals attack from a sense of frustration, but whatever the reason, the danger remains.

Approaching animals

As was noted under the heading of behaviour, an animal judges the nature of its response to the approach of a man by his actions.   If he talks soothingly, and moves slowly and firmly without jerks, the animal will not get nervous and will be less afraid and more easily handled.   The necessity for restraint varies with each animal species, but in respect to cattle the most common requirement is that the animal be held for examination.   This may be done by a rope around the horns, or better, by the use of a halter.   Bulls are always potentially dangerous, and should have a ring put in the nose so that the head can be controlled with a bull pole. Bull-dogs or bull-holders should only be used in cattle when other methods of holding the head have failed.

    Cows commonly prod with their horns, or kick forward (cow kick) with their hooves, although occasional cows in byres or standings have learnt to kick backwards.   Many have an annoying habit of squeezing a person wishing to reach their heads against the side of the stall.   Bulls should always be held by a bull pole and, if a crush is not available, be put in a three pole holder for examination.   With modern sedatives and tranquilizers there is no need to fight an animal

RESTRAINT OF CATTLE

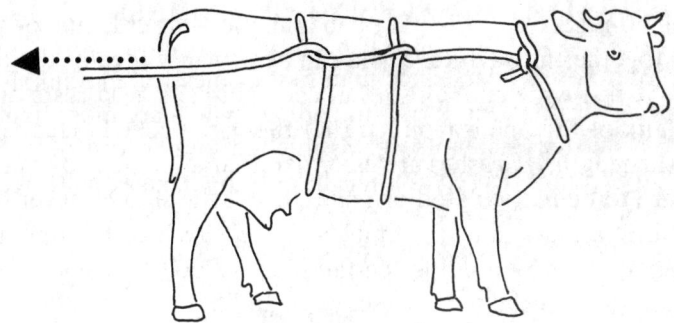

Method of Casting a Cow

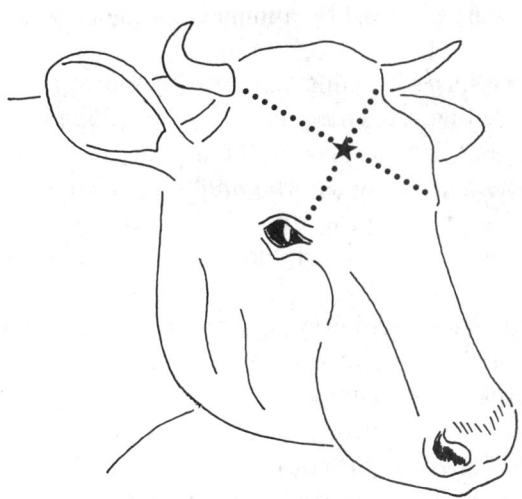

Aiming Point When Shooting Cattle

Figure 42

in order to examine it.   It is far better to use a modern drug and to do the job properly; the use of xylazine in the correct dose enables cattle to be examined standing.

Use of crushers

A crush consists of a collecting pen and a long double line of poles bound together into which cattle can be driven.   Ideally the crush should be just wide enough so that each animal's head rests on the right flank of the one is front so that they are packed diagonally along the length.   Crushes are essential if large number of ranch cattle are to be innoculated or marked.   Cattle should never be beaten into a crush; a lead animal is pushed towards the opening and lead along it by holding the tail high.   Good herdsmen will see that the others in the pen can see it go and are able to follow it into the crush one by one.   Each animal is packed against the one in front by raising the tail and guiding it forward.   Young calves should never be introduced with older animals, deaths in crushes are all caused by small animals being trampled by those behind.   Great care is needed to see that the front animal is not crushed against the opening bars.   Single animal by animal crushes can be made for dairy cows.

If it can be avoided, restraint of a cow for the carrying out of a painful or frightening procedure should not be done in the stall in which it is milked.   Disturbance in the milking stall leads to a drop in milk yield and nervousness during milking which will take some time to pass.   No painful procedure should take place without local or general anaesthetic, and all should be carried out by a veterinary surgeon.

The illustration shows an easy way to cast a cow or ox.   It consists of a continuous series of rope loops leading from the neck, passing round the thorax behind the foreleg, and in front of the udder.   It seems to be the pressure on the last loop which causes the ox to lie down.   Even a light cord pulled tight around the body in the region of the udder will stop a cow kicking.

If cattle are cast they should not be allowed to remain on their sides for any length of time since gas will form in the rumen and they will become blown.   As many procedures as possible should be carried out while the animal is standing.

Restraint of dogs

It is only proposed to mention one method of restraint in dogs, that is the technique of tying a bandage round the jaws to prevent the animal biting.   Two loops are made in the bandage, and one is twisted in placing it onto the first loop.   This is slipped over the jaws and drawn tight, the ends being tied behind the head below the ears.

If there is any suspicion of rabies then the dog should be caught in a dog-catcher.   This consists of a pole with a strong ring at the end, the rope runs through a metal loop fixed into the pole 22 cm (9 in) from its end and fastened to the end ring.   The loop of rope between the end ring and the metal loop is then passed over the dog's head and drawn tight while holding the pole firmly.

GENERAL NURSING OF ANIMALS

There are very many things that can be done to help an animal to recover from an accident or the results of a disease, which do not include the use of specific medicines.   Careful nursing will often bring an animal back to health when all the medicines that have been thought of have failed.

Protection from weather

No ruminant animal, that is ox, sheep or goat, should be left on its side, this is particularly important in the case of cattle.   It must be laid, with its head up, on the brisket and the legs arranged under it in the natural way.   It may be propped up in the right position with sacks or bales.

An animal which is down must be protected from the weather. This means providing shade from the sun, cover from rain, and shelter from wind depending on the climate.   Most important, it should be given as much clean water to drink as it requires.   If it is down for more than a few hours it must be moved regularly from one side to the other.   Cows which are down for more than two days are often very difficult to raise, probably because they are nervous about their ability to stand.   If there is no known cause for them continuing to lie down, then they ought to be persuaded to stand, and supported

once they have done so, until the feeling has returned to their legs.
If a cow can be persuaded to rise and can be supported for a few
minutes in a standing position it will be seen to get its confidence
back, and will gradually take its own balance.   The longer a cow is
down the longer it will take to recover.

Sometimes a cow will stay down after a bad calving; this is caused
by pressure damage of the calf on the main nerves to the hind legs.
The same principle applies; the sooner the cow rises the better and as
soon as it has overcome its exhaustion attempts should be made to
raise it.   Except in the case of very valuable animals it is hardly worth
persisting with an animal which has been down after calving for more
than five days.   On the fifth day therefore help should be sought to
raise the animal by all possible means, including bodily raising it and
putting it on its feet.   If this fails then it should be slaughtered.
When cows become recumbent in a tropical climate where the temperature and humidity are high it is rarely worth persisting with efforts
to get them to stand, beyond the third day.

Cattle are calmer if they can see their companions, and it is better
to nurse a cow in a pen with an open side where it can see other cattle.
Adequate food must be brought to it.   Green sweet grass or concentrates should be fed until the animal rejoins the herd.   The pen
should be cleaned out regularly and clean bedding provided.

The consistency of the dung should be examined carefully, if the
animal is constipated and losing condition then look to see whether
it is getting sufficient water.   A rise of temperature may mean an
infection, and the most frequent source of this is either the calfbed
in a newly calved cow or the lungs.   In either case there may be a
case for considering antibiotics.

The signs of returning health are pinkness of the mucous membranes
of the eye, greater alertness and curiosity and normal temperature.
Signs of declining health are movement over the eye of the third eyelid, high temperature, foetid discharge, and rasping breathing.

There is a look of complete disinterest in the eye of a dying animal.
It is lethargic and makes little effort to help itself.   The ears droop,
and the head and tail are unsupported.   The body temperature drops
shortly before death and frequently there is relaxation of the sphincter
muscles resulting in urination.

THE SLAUGHTER AND DESTRUCTION OF ANIMALS

Animals are fortunate that they do not appear to anticipate death. Of course one of their survival mechanisms is to avoid those situations which are likely to result in injury, and which by experience they know to be painful. In considering our human attitude to the destruction of animals it is as well to bear in mind these and other considerations.

The reasons why animals are slaughtered

Man is an omnivore but he has a taste preference for animal protein. Some people choose not to eat meat, and some people have no access to it, but the fact remains that man is dependent on the destruction of animals for an essential part of his diet. Human populations are now so large that enormous numbers of animals have to be destroyed each day throughout the world in order to meet this need. While one must respect the views of people who abhor this situation, nevertheless one must also recognize that it is not going to be changed in the foreseeable future. At the present time there is no substitute food available which can replace meat in the human diet. For various reasons, milk and eggs are not entirely acceptable to many communities even if they could be produced in sufficient quantity to make possible the avoidance of meat eating.

Destruction of animals would in any case take place regardless of the fact that they are to be eaten. The land mass of the world is just not large enough to support animals, as well as man, to the limit of both their life spans. Having accepted that the destruction of animals is a necessity, we have an equal responsibility to see that it is carried out with the least possible distress to the animal.

The fact of death

It is accepted that the brain is the repository of man's and animal's conscious knowledge of the environment. Cessation of the ability of the brain to function results in a permanent interruption of the receipt of messages along the brain trunks of the body. There can therefore be no appreciation of pain because the animal has become unconscious.

The cells in the tissues continue to live for a time after their blood supply is cut off by the failure of the heart, although heart beats continue for some time after brain destruction. With the failure of circulation the cells in the tissues die progressively in inverse proportion to their dependence on oxygen. The more organized cells require more oxygen than the simpler cellular elements.

It is of interest to compare the results of killing an animal by inducing a failure of blood circulation and by destruction of the brain. In most hunting situations a heart shot is used, the object being to disrupt the major vessels at the point where they leave the ventricles. Even when the shot is completely accurate the animal often runs for up to 30 m; a similar type of effect is seen when the major vessels of the neck are severed. There is activity for an appreciable time thereafter, and that activity tends to be coordinated. That is the animal is capable of running or struggling, both actions requiring central coordination. This does not happen with brain destruction, any subsequent movement is incoordinated and therefore due to reflex actions originating in the lower regions of the vertebral column. The hunted animal shot through the brain falls instantly to the ground.

There can remain little doubt therefore, in the thoughtful observer's mind, that slaughter ought to be practiced by destruction of the brain. At this point the animal is dead in the sense that it can have no conscious knowledge of what is happening to its body.

The responsibility of man in animal destruction

We cannot avoid destroying animals but we can avoid distressing them in doing so. Confusion and noises are the factors which cause animals great distress, and by observation the sight of blood and offal do not affect animals in the way they affect man. This is probably because man automatically transposes a situation seen into a possible prediction of injury to himself. In short, human beings experience shock in seeing injury because they imagine what it must be like to suffer the same injury themselves. It is however evident that even the most sensitive people, in the presence of the spectacular results of injury, become rapidly hardened, and learn to cut imagination short. Otherwise the work of doctors, nurses, and others involved in emergency services would be impossible. All the evidence points to the fact that animals do not have this sort of imagination. Left to themselves in a slaughter house, and without the pressure of herding and noise, they will wander among carcases quite undisturbed by the implications.

The first criteria of humane slaughter are therefore calm, quiet, organized, and unflustered surroundings. There should be no shouting; where possible animals should be lead and not driven. Cattle are certainly calmer when water is being sprinkled upon them, and since this also helps in making an electrical contact, this has a useful purpose in an organized meat processing factory. When individual animals are being destroyed the attitude of the person doing it is very important; if he is calm the animal will be unworried, if he is aggressive the animal will return the aggression.

Humane slaughter of food animals

The second important point is that consciousness should be destroyed as quickly as possible. For quick humane slaughter there is no substitute for a humane killer applied in the right place on the head so that the captive bolt or the bullet will destroy the brain. The usual procedure is to shoot the animal and then introduce a steel rod through the hole and into the spinal cord, so destroying the nervous tissue. If the animal has been electrocuted it is, in the view of the author, essential that it should also be shot in the way described. It is quite impossible to form a judgement on whether electrocuted animals are immobilized or unconscious. The balance of evidence indicates the latter, however it is a subject which should not be open to debate.

The point at which to aim varies with each species of animal. In the ox it is not between the eyes but at the point where two imaginary lines drawn between each eye and each opposite ear crosses. There is often a whorl of hair at this point which can be a guide. In pigs the point is rather higher than the line of the eyes and to one side of the strong saggital crest which arises in this region. In sheep the same principles apply as in cattle. Many communities in the tropics are extremely skilled in killing cattle or buffalo by pithing, that is by severing the spinal cord at the back of the neck between the skull and the first neck vertebra.   In the hands of a skilled herdsman this is extremely effective, very humane, and probably kinder to the animal than the procedure in many European slaughter houses.

All food animals are bled as soon as possible after death.   This is achieved by severing the jugular and carotid arteries, usually on the left side, and as close as possible to the chest cavity.   Bleeding is said to improve the keeping quality of the meat and may be a survival from biblical times when animals were killed in hot climates without the benefits of refrigeration.   Certainly nowadays it enables a valuable by-product to be collected.

The destruction of pet animals

Destruction by shooting is not a satisfactory method in dogs and cats; not only is it aesthetically unacceptable, but it is not a precise enough method in unskilled hands.   Anaesthetic and immobilizing drugs are now freely available and can ensure that the animal is under no stress when the time comes to end its life.   Two anaesthetics in common use are concentrated pentobarbitone in dogs and cats, and etorphine in dogs.   The former given intravenously or intraperitoneally and the latter intramuscularly.   Both have the effect of inducing sleep, although it may be necessary to use other agents once the animal is unconscious.

In countries where rabies is prevalent there is no substitute for the use of a shotgun on suspect cases out of doors.   Heavy shot of grade SSG is usually used, and destruction is painless, and without risk to the operator.

Destruction of horses

When other means are not available then the shooting of horses when carried out by skilled hands is the most satisfactory method of destruction.   It is probably best carried out with a special bell-shaped adaptor with a wide mouth, and provision for a cartridge at its apex. This is placed on the head and fires a low velocity bullet into the brain.   Unless the person is a skilled marksman, and entirely familiar with the weapon, revolvers should never be used to destroy horses, and under no circumstances should they be used in a closed box.   A shotgun using heavy shot (SSG) is very satisfactory provided that the horse is held in the open air, the aiming point is on the side of the head just below the line of the eye and ear and slightly upwards across the head.   It is, however, a method for an emergency.   A number of anaesthetic agents can be used in the horse.   The most obvious and the most effective being concentrated pentobartitone given intravenously in high dose.   Barbiturates cannot, of course, be used in animals intended for human food.

One point should be made in regard to the destruction of pet horses.   It is always advisable to consider the means of disposal of the carcase before destroying the animal.   Physically the hardest part of the operation is digging the grave.   This is best left to the owner despite the fact that many owners underestimate the size of the task in the emotion of the moment.

Appendix 1

Glossary

Abomasum: True stomach of the ruminant, leading into the small intestine.

Acaricide: Substance which kills mites.

Acetabulum: Joint between the pelvis and femur on the hind leg.

Acetonaemia: A failure of metabolism in the dairy cow, characterized by the presence of sweet smelling ketone bodies in the breath.

Adjuvant: Substance, which, when mixed with an antigen, improves the response to a vaccine.

Aldosterone: The main mineralocorticoid excreted by the adrenal cortex. It influences the balance of electrolytes in the body.

Adrenal gland: Gland lying close to the kidneys.

Adrenaline: Selectively stimulates sympathetic nerves. It increases heart beat, increases wakefulness and respiration, reduces appetite. It stimulates the metabolism increasing the use of oxygen, and increases blood sugar. It affects smooth muscle selectively, increasing activity in the skin and decreasing it in the intestine.

Allergy: Hypersensitive reaction of the body to a protein which it has encountered on a previous occasion. The allergy usually takes the form of a rash but signs of shock may be seen in extreme cases.

Alveolae: The air sac at the end of the bronchioles in the lungs, on the surface of which oxygen/carbon dioxide exchange takes place.

Analgesic: A substance which relieves pain.

Anaphylaxis: Similar to allergy but more severe in reaction. The cause, as in allergy, is the acute inter-reaction of antigen and antibody which results in a shock-like reaction.

Androgen: A male sex hormone, either natural or synthesized.

Anoestrus: The period of inactivity in the female sexual cycle, its most obvious manifestation is in animals of the canine species.

Anoxia: State of deprivation of oxygen.

Anthelmintic: Remedy active against helminth parasites.

194

Antibody: Substance produced by the body to counter a specific antigen.

Antigen: A substance, usually a protein, which produces a specific antibody in response to its introduction into the blood stream.

Aorta: The main artery conveying blood from the left ventricle to the body.

Arteries: Vessels which convey blood from the ventricles to the body.

Arterioles: The smallest arteries which branch into capillaries in the tissues.

Auricle: The vessels in which the blood collects before passing through valves into the heart ventricles.

Axon: The filament of the nerve cell along which messages pass to and from the tissues.

Babesia: Protozoal parasites living, and multiplying in red blood cells.

Bactericidal: A substance which will kill bacteria. It is usually applied to the actions of antibiotics in the body. Penicillin and streptomycin are both bacteriocidal.

Bacteriostatic: A substance which prevents bacteria multiplying. It is usually applied to antibiotics which have this action within the body. Tetracyclines are bacteriostatic in action.

Bile duct: The duct conveying bile from the liver to the intestine.

Biologicals: Vaccines.

Bloat: Distension of the rumen in cattle, and other ruminants, arising from uncontrolled fermentation of the ruminal contents.

B.P.C.: The British Pharmaceutical Codex which lists the substances used in medicine, their actions, and dosage recommendations.

Broilers: Intensively reared hybrid chickens capable of effective food conversion and rapid growth. They are usually slaughtered at about 9 weeks of age at 1·75 kg (4 lb) in weight.

Bronchioles: The small air ducts found in the lungs which connect the bronchi and the alveolae.

Caecum: A closed intestinal tube lying between the small and large intestines, usually well developed in herbivores, and vestigial in carnivores.

Canines: Animals of the dog family with distinctive eye teeth.

Capillaries: The network of small blood vessels joining the arteries and veins within the tissues.

Carbohydrate: Starchy organic food broken down into water and energy in the body.

Carnassial teeth: The modified cheek teeth found in carnivores and used for cutting tissues by a scissor action.

Carnivore: An animal dependent upon other animal tissues for its food.

Carpal bones: The small bones between the radius and ulna and the metacarpals.

Cellular immunity: Immunity which is contained within the cells of the body, and in particular the macrophages, or scavenging cells. It permits them to digest invading organisms, and stimulates them to seek out foreign proteins entering the body.

Cerebellum: That area of the brain which coordinates movement.

Cerebrum: That area of the brain where the recognition of the environment is located, and where response to external stimuli are directed.

Cervical: Found in the neck, and applied to vertebrae in that region.

Cervix: The muscular sphincter found between the uterus and the vagina in the reproductive tract.

Cestodes: Helminths of the tapeworm family. They have a complex life history involving entry into secondary hosts which are often the victims of the final host, or are ingested by the final host.

Chalaza: The twisted membrane which suspends the yolk in the white in the eggs of birds.

Chemotherapeutic: A chemical substance which is produced for use in medicine. It is very loosely applied to all chemicals used in treatment which do not fall into well recognized categories.

Chorionic gonadotrophin: This is a hormone obtained from the urine of pregnant women, and originating in the chorion or lining of the placenta. It is luteinizing hormone, or LH, of value in obtaining the release of the ovum from the mature ovarian follicle.

Clavicle: The shoulder bone. It is known as the wishbone in chickens.

Cloaca: The combined opening for urine and faeces in birds.

Clostridia: A family of sporulating, anaerobic, Gram-positive, bacteria responsible for many diseases in animals. The effects of the disease are produced by exotoxins.

Coccidiostat: A substance which prevent coccidia multiplying in the intestinal wall.

Coccygeal: Appertaining to the coccyx or tail.

Coitus: Sexual copulation.

Colon: The large intestine between the point at which the caecum emerges and the rectum.

Colostrum: The yellow coloured milk produced immediately after parturition, and rich in immuno-globulins.

Convoluted tubule: The many coiled knot of blood vessels in the glomerulus of the kidney where excretion of water and other substances takes place.

Coracoid: The bone joining the sternum and the vertebrae in birds.

Corpus luteum: The yellow body which results after the rupture of the ovarian follicle at oestrus. It persists for varying periods in different species of animals, and excretes progesterone.

Cortex: The outer area of an organ, commonly applied to the kidneys and adrenals where there is an obvious division into outer cortical zone and inner medullary zone. Both zones have different functions in both organs.

Corticosteroids: Substances excreted by the cortex of the adrenal gland which provide the chemical regulation of metabolism in the body. Synthetic corticosteroids have similar but enhanced activity.

Cranium: The case of bone which encompasses the brain.

Defaecation: The act of discharge of waste matter from the rectum through the anus.

Dehydration: The act of losing water from the body. It may occur from perspiration but is the term commonly used to denote the loss of water in extreme diarrhoea. It is this loss of water from the tissues and the failure of the body to correct the flow which is so lethal in cases of dysentery.

Dermatological: Appertaining to the skin.

Diabetes: There are two types of diabetes. Diabetes mellitus is produced by a failure in the secretion of insulin from the pancreas. It is characterized by high blood sugar levels. Diabetes insipidus is the term given to frequent urination caused by a failure in the secretion of a hormone which controls the excretion of water through the kidneys.

Diaphragm: The large combined muscle and tendon which divides the chest or thorax from the abdomen. Not found in birds.

Diurnal: Occurring during the day.

Drug resistance: The property of certain bacteria and protozoa to develop resistance against drugs which would otherwise destroy them. Inherited drug resistance refers to the property, recently discovered, where the resistance which has been developed by one species of bacteria, may be conveyed to quite dissimilar organisms by transfer of genetic material.

Drying off: Term applied when stopping milking a dairy cow in the weeks before the next parturition or calving.

Ductus deferens: The duct along which sperm travel during ejaculation by the male animal.

Electrolyte: Any substance which conducts electricity with the production of a gas or a solid at one of the electrodes.

Embryo: The early stage of growth of multicellular animals after fertilization of the egg by the sperm.

Endotoxins: The name given to organic poisons conveyed by the bodies of bacteria which produce them.

Epididymis: The body lying above the testicles, and containing the tiny tubules which lead from the seminal cells of the testes. They join together to form the ductus deferens, and they act as collection vehicles for the sperm.

Epiglottis: The leaf-like structure at the back of the mouth which protects the entrance to the lungs when food is being swallowed.

Faeces: Waste products evacuated from the rectum through the anus.

Fallopian tube: The tube along which ova travel on their way to the uterus.

False pregnancy: The appearance of signs indicating pregnancy despite the bitch having failed to conceive at oestrus. The commonest signs consist of nervousness and milk production. They are only found in the presence of a corpus luteum.

Femur: The first long bone of the hind leg.

Fetus: The young animal between the embryo stage and birth.

Fibrinogen: A protein found in blood plasma, which combined with thrombin from platelets produces fibrin, the basic component of clots.

Foramen: A hole in a bone through which veins, arteries and nerves pass. On occasion it describes circular openings in bones which rest upon other bones. In essence a window.

Formalin: A shortened word form of formaldehyde, which, in 10% solution is used to preserve pathological specimens.

FSH: Follicle stimulating hormone, the means by which ovarian follicles are stimulated to develop to maturity. It is serum gonadotrophin in the commercial form, and is obtained from the blood of mares in early pregnancy.

Galactophore: The opening of the teat duct at the bottom of the teat through which milk is drawn by the young animal. The number of galactophores per teat varies in different species of animals.

Germinal disk: The small conglomeration of cells which will feed upon the yolk in the eggs of birds, and develop into an embryo.

Gestation period: The period of pregnancy which precedes parturition.

Gilt: Female pig before its first litter, sometimes up to the birth of the second litter.

Glomerulus: The conglomeration of cells in the cortex of the kidney responsible for the secretion of nitrogen from the body.

Glycogen: Animal starch, it is stored in the liver, and utilized when glucose is required to meet energy requirements.

Gram-negative: Gram was a Dutch scientist working in the twentiety century who developed a stain to distinguish certain types of bacteria. Gram-negative bacteria are those which are decolorized by alcohol after they have been stained by Gram's stain.

Gram-positive: Bacteria not decolorized with alcohol after staining with Gram's stain.

Growth stimulant: A substance which, added to the diet of intensively reared animals will improve their growth rate. It is possible that the effect is due to control of sub-clinical infections of intestinal bacteria.

Haemoglobin: The substance which conveys oxygen and carbon dioxide around the body by loose attachment. It is present in red blood cells and gives them their distinctive colour.

Haematocytoblast: The precursor cell of red blood cells found in bone marrow.

Heifer: Female bovine either up to the age of puberty, or to the time of the first calf, occasionally up to the time of the second calf.

Helminth: The term applied to parasitic worms of the biological phyla Platyhelminthes (flukes, tapeworms and flatworms) and Nematheminthes (roundworms and associated forms). Hence helminthology is the study of all varieties of parasitic worms.

Herbivore: An animal which depends for its food entirely on plant tissues.

Humoral immunity: That type of immune response which circulates in the body fluids. It consists of specific antibodies produced in response to specific antigens.

Humerus: First long bone of the arm or foreleg.

Ileum: The posterior end of the small intestine immediately before it joins the large intestine.

Ilium: Part of the pelvic girdle of the skeleton.

Immobilizing agent: A substance which when injected into an animal prevents it using its voluntary muscles. It is not necessarily an anaesthetic, but the difference between one and the other is sometimes difficult to establish particularly where animals are concerned.

Immunity: The defences that an animal acquires with the experience of overcoming organisms or biological substances which cause disease.

Immuno-globulins: Complex proteins which carry protective antibodies.

Incisors: The front teeth prominent in rodents.

Inguinal groove: The channel or opening in the abdominal cavity, lined with peritoneum, through which the spermatic chord passes.

Insulin: A substance excreted by the pancreas which influences glucose concentration in the blood.

In vitro: The term used to describe the observed action of a chemotherapeutic or biological substance outside the body.

In vivo: Similar action but observed by reactions occurring inside the body, usually of experimental animals.

Keratin: The material, largely composed of dead epithelial skin cells, which accumulates on the surface of the skin. Strictly speaking it should be applied to dead cells excreted by the body.

Larynx: The complex organ, composed of muscle and cartilage, lying at the top of the trachea, and responsible for voice and sound production.

Leucocyte: A white blood cell.

LH: Luteinizing hormone.

Ligament: The fibrous attachment of muscles to bones.

Lumbar: Term applied to the region in the middle of the back.

Lymph: A fluid resembling blood plasma which circulates in the tissue spaces, and which contains numerous lymphocytes.

Lymphatic system: The system which contains lymph and which ensures its circulation round the body.

Lymphocyte: A small white cell found throughout the body, and which is probably the repository of most of the body's immune reactions.

Lysis: The act of destruction of cells, commonly applied to red blood cells, which when lysed release haemoglobin which colours the fluid in which they are circulating.

Malpighian capsules: The secretory body found in numbers in the kidneys and which are responsible for nitrogen secretion.

Mandible: Lower jaw.

Mastitis: Inflammation of the udder.

Mediastinal glands: Lymph glands found in the chest or thorax and lying in the fibrous tissue known as the mediastinum, which suspends the organs of the chest.

Medulla oblongata: The terminal portion of the brain which extends into the spinal column.

Mendelian laws: A number of laws of 'nature' devised by a monk called Mendel as a result of his experiments on the inheritance of characters in living animals. He discovered that some inherited characteristics are dominant, and some recessive, so that the characteristics found in the young are never merely a simple mixture of those of their parents.

Meninges: The fibrous covering of the brain and spinal cord.

Mesenteric glands: Lymph glands found in the abdomen and associated with the mesentery or suspensory tissue of the abdominal organs.

Metacarpal: The terminal bones of the front limb.

Metatarsal: The terminal bones of the hind limb.

Metoestrus: The time in the female cycle coming after oestrus, and before ano-estrus or dioestrus, in the absence of pregnancy.

Molars: The cheek or grinding teeth.

Myeloid tissue: The blood cell producing tissue of the long bone marrow.

Necrosis: The result of the destruction of tissue within the body.

Nematodes: Members of the biological phylum Nemathelminthes or roundworms.

Neonate: Animal at the time of its emergence from its mother's uterus.

Neuron: Nerve cell.

Nocturnal: Night operating

Nidation: The implantation of the fertilized ovum in the lining of the uterus in the first stage of pregnancy.

Oesophagus: That part of the digestive tract lying between the pharynx and the stomach.

Oestrogen: Hormones associated with the production of female characteristics.

Oestrus: Period in the sexual cycle when the female will accept the male.

Omasum: The third stomach of the ruminant which functions as a mixing organ for the food substances.

Organic compounds: Substances containing carbon.

Ovariohysterectomy: Removal of the ovary and uterus in the female. Often referred to as spaying.

Ovulation: The extrusion of the ovum from the follicle at the climax of the sexual cycle.

Pancreas: A large elongated gland found in the loop of the duodenum (a part of the small intestine). It has two functions. It aids digestion by secreting four enzymes (amylopsin, trypsin, steapsin and rennin) into the duodenum. It also releases insulin into the blood stream so controlling glucose metabolism.

Parturition: Act of giving birth.

Patella: Knee bone.

Pathology: The study of the effects of disease on organs and tissues. Hence pathogenic substances are those which damage tissues and organs.

Pericardium: The suspensory ligament of the heart.

Peristalsis: The rhythmic movements of the intestine which drives food along the digestive tract.

Peritoneum: The tissue lining the abdomen and abdominal organs.

Pessary: Preparation placed in the vagina.

Phagocytes: White cells which engulf invasive organisms.

Phalanges: The digits.

Plasma: The liquid in which the blood cells circulate.

Pleural cavities: The cavities, one each side of the chest, in which the lungs lie.

PMS: Pregnant Mare Serum—a commercial source of follicle stimulating hormone or FSH.

Premunition: A state of resistance to parasitic disease which is dependant on the presence of small numbers of the parasite in the body.

Progestagen: Commercially available substances with the same, but enhanced properties, as natural progesterone.

Progesterone: The hormone which, in general terms, maintains pregnancy.

Prolactin: The hormone which stimulates milk production in the pregnant animal.

Prophylaxis: The use of substances which enhance the body's capacity to resist disease.

Pro-oestrus: That part of the sexual cycle which precedes oestrus.

Protoplasm: The only known form in which life exists. It is a substance bound in a jelly like form by water, and it contains proteins, lipins (fatty substances) carbohydrates and inorganic salts.

Ptyalin: Enzyme secreted by the salivary glands to assist the digestion of starch.

Pygostyle: The bone at the end of the vertebral column of birds.

Radius: One of the bones of the forelimb lying between the carpals and the humerus.

Reflex action: An action which has become imprinted on the brain and which is coordinated without conscious thought.

Reticulum: The second stomach of the ruminant which has a characteristic honeycomb lining.

Retina: The light sensitive lining of the eyeball.

Rickettsia: Micro-organisms considered to lie, in the biological classification scale, between bacteria and viruses. They are responsible for some dangerous diseases and are frequently transmitted by ticks.

Rumen: The first and most capacious stomach of the ruminant. It acts as a storage organ for vegetable matter, where bacteria can break down the cellulose, and from which it can be regurgitated for further chewing.

Sacrum: The fused bones of the vertebral column lying just in front of the pelvis.

Sclera: The fibrous lining of the eye.

Sedative: A drug which reduces the activity of the brain, and therefore lowers the level of response to external stimuli.

Serum: The blood fluid when cells and the material responsible for clots has been removed. Plasma without cells and after clotting.

Serum gonadotrophin: see PMS.

Synergism: The effect of two drugs acting together to produce an action of greater intensity than would be possible by the sum of both their actions assessed separately.

Therapeutic index: The ratio between the curative and toxic dose of a drug used in the treatment of animals and man.

Tranquillizer: Drugs which, when given to man, make him indifferent to his surroundings. It is by no means clear whether they have similar effects in animals.

Trematodes: Parasitic worms of the biological class Trematoda of the phylum Platyhelminthes. Usually known as flukes.

Tympanites: Bloat.

Ulna: The bone lying next to the radius in the forelimb.

Urea: The last breakdown product of protein in the body, and the means by which nitrogen is excreted. It has been synthesized and fed to cattle in nitrogen deficient areas of the world, and in the dry season. It cannot be overfed.

Ventricle: A chamber, usually reserved for the description of the muscular chambers in the heart responsible for the blood circulation.

Zoonosis: A disease which affects man and animals.

Appendix 2

Useful Information

Some average life spans of animals

Name of animal	Years	Name of animal	Years
Bear	30	Horse	20
Cat	12	Lion	25
Cow	20	Monkey	15
Dog	10	Parrot	30
Dove	15	Rabbit	12
Elephant	60	Rat	3
Goat	15	Sheep	12
Goose	30	Tiger	20

Constituents of normal milk

Species	Water %	Fat %	Protein %	Lactose %	Ash %
Bitch	78·88	8·56	6·82	4·09	0·51
Buffalo	82·55	7·12	4·15	4·99	0·865
Cow	87·25	3·80	3·50	4·80	0·65
Ewe	80·82	6·86	6·52	4·91	0·89
Goat	87·3	3·9	3·5	4·5	0·8
Mare	90·70	1·20	2·00	5·70	0·40
Sow	84·09	4·56	7·23	3·13	1·05
Human	80·30	3·11	1·19	7·18	0·21

Table of oestrous cycle, age of puberty etc., in domesticated animals.

	Cow	Mare	Buffalo	Ewe	Goat	Sow	Bitch
Age of puberty	24–36 months	12–24 months	24–36 months	8–12 months	8–12 months	4–6 months	5–6 months
Length of oestrous cycle	18–24 days	14–21 days	21 days (variable)	15–19 days	18–21 days	1 day	6 months
Duration of heat	4–20 hours	2–6 days	36 hours	36 hours	24–36 hours	2–3 days	9–18 days
Time of ovulation	14 hours after oestrus	24–48 hours before end of oestrus	—	24–48 hours after onset of oestrus	—	35 hours after onset of oestrus	2 days after coitus
Gestation period	280 days	336 days	300 days	150 days	150 days	114 days	60 days
Return of heat after parturition	30–60 days	3–4 weeks	30–60 days	3 weeks	3 weeks	2 months	16 weeks
Age of weaning	8–16 weeks	12–16 weeks	12–16 weeks	8–16 weeks	6–10 weeks	3–6 weeks	4–6 weeks

Numbers of mammary glands and of galactophores (teat ducts) occurring in some domestic and laboratory species of animals

Species	No. of mammary glands	No. of galactophores per teat
Cat	4 pairs	4–7
Cow	Udder has (4 quarters)	1
Goat	Udder has (2 halves)	1
Sheep	Udder has (2 halves)	1
Dog	5 pairs	8–20
Guinea pig	1 pair	1
Mare	1 pair	2–4
Mouse	5 pairs	1
Pig	5–6 pairs	2–3
Rabbit	4–5 pairs	8–10
Rat	6 pairs	1

Metrication guide

Length

1 centimetre	(cm) =	0·394 inch
1 metre	(m) =	1·0936 yards
1 kilometre	(km) =	0·6214 mile—roughly 1·6 km = 1 mile
1 square km	(km^2) =	0·3861 square mile
1 hectare	(ha) =	2·4711 acres—roughly 2·5 acres = 1 ha

Weight

1 gram	(g) =	0·0353 oz
1 kilogram	(kg) =	2·2046 lb
1 tonne	(t) =	1·1023 short tons or 0·9842 ton (Avoirdupois)
1 ton (Avoirdupois)	=	1·0161 tonne (t)—a metric tonne and an avoirdupois ton are the same for most practical purposes

Volume and capacity

1 ml	(cc) =	1000th of a litre
1 litre	=	1$\frac{3}{4}$ pts = 0·2200 gal. Between 4$\frac{1}{2}$ & 4·6 litres = 1 gal.
1 cubic metre	(m^3) =	roughly 220 gals.

Pulse, respirations and temperature

	Pulse beats/min	Respirations/ min	Temperature F°	C°
Horse	38–43	8–12	100–101	37·8–38·3
Cow	50–60	12–16	101–102	38·3–38·9
Sheep	75–80	20–30	103–104	39·4–40·0
Pig	70–80	20–30	102–103	38·9–39·4
Dog	80–90	15–25	101–102	38·3–38·9
Cat	150–200	20–40	101–102	38·3–38·9

Index

X